THE REAL PFIZER PAPERS

A. LE ROY

UNPARAGONED

Formatted with Vellum

BATTLE MANUALS FOR FREEDOM

GENI.US/RIGHTS

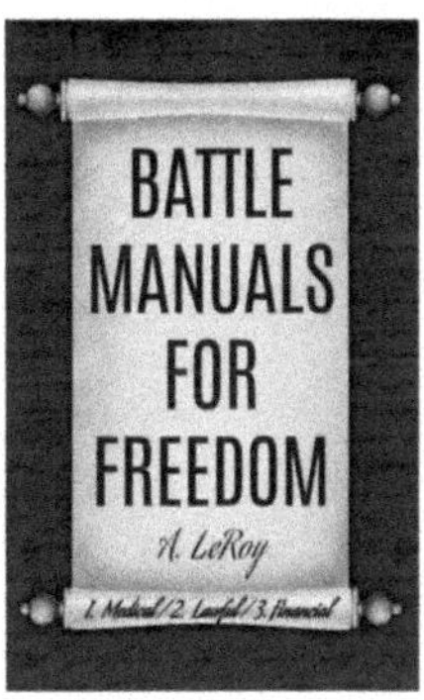

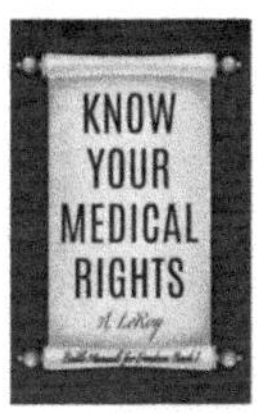

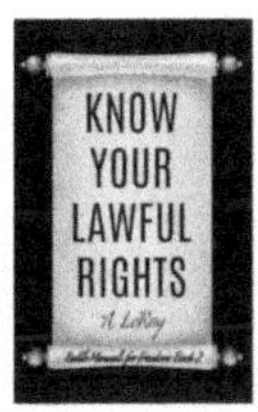

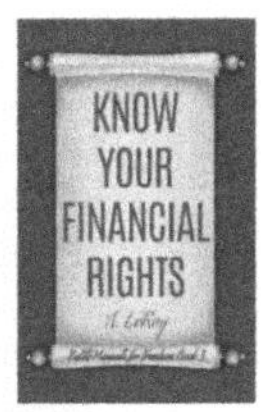

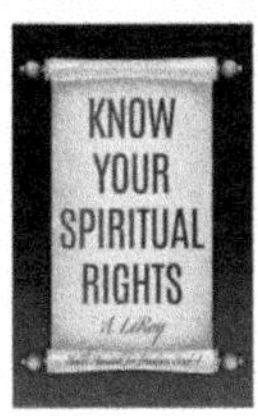

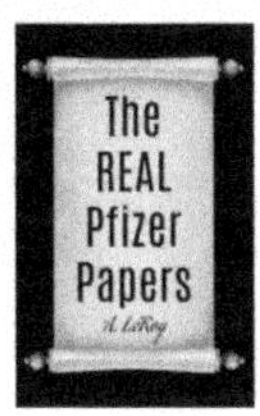

Book 1: *Know Your Medical Rights*

Book 2: *Know Your Lawful Rights*

Book 3: *Know Your Financial Rights*

Book 4: *Know Your Spiritual Rights*

CONTENTS

INTRODUCTION

For a while, I was Controlled Opposition, but I didn't know it at the time...

In the Spring of 2022, I began working for a law firm that has won acclaim in the so-called 'Medical-Freedom Movement'. One of my tasks was to investigate the clinical-trial papers Pfizer had sent to the FDA to get its COVID 'vaccine' licensed.

Widely known as the 'Pfizer Papers', these documents were prised from regulators by legal process after the FDA tried to spread their release over several decades. They are available for anyone to download at https://phmpt.org/pfizer-16-plus-documents, but as they comprise hundreds of thousands of pages across hundreds of files in varying formats, all released at different times, and when they sometimes resort to impenetrable scientific jargon and include redactions, the Papers are not exactly accessible to your average reader.

To turn all that raw information into something useful and coherent, I sifted carefully through the entire collection, sometimes combining the files into huge PDF or Word files in order to run searches for various terms. In the process, I found nuggets that Naomi Wolf had missed in her book, *The Pfizer Papers: Pfizer's Crimes Against Humanity*, which she compiled in cooperation with the DailyClout team of investigative volunteers. I found, for example, that...

- Pfizer acknowledged to the FDA that its 'vaccine' trials in adolescents were illegally premature. These were the trials, conducted by Dr. Robert Frenck at Cincinnatti Children's Hospital, that put 12-year-old Maddie de Garay in a wheelchair and on a feeding tube. Yet Frenck would go on to claim, in a *New England Journal of Medicine* article of May 27, 2021 that Pfizer's vaccine "had a favorable safety and side-effect profile... There were no vaccine-related serious adverse events and few overall severe adverse events" (p.1, p.239).

- The Pfizer papers included resumes of the investigators conducting clinical trials for its COVID 'vaccine'. The vast majority had signed their resumes in the Spring and Summer of

2020, consistent with the timing of those trials, but 13 investigators had signed in 2018 and 2019. Was Pfizer lining them up before this novel disease had even appeared?

- Pfizer had been in talks with the FDA about injecting newborns, not just the six-month-olds reached on June 17, 2022 after the FDA had issued a series of 'emergency-use authorizations' (EUA) to younger and younger age groups.

I shared my findings with my main contact at the law firm, but when I pointed out the illegality of Pfizer's adolescent trials, her answer made no sense. It felt like she was was trying to explain it away. I remember thinking at the time, "Are you working for Pfizer?"

Still, I pressed on with my task and wrote a series of 17 articles based on my findings, until the firm informed me by email in August 2023 that they would not use them and to "cease doing work for the firm." I was fired from my freelance role, albeit in a lawerly way, but had permission to use the articles in my own name.

Here they are in this book. Perhaps you will find them helpful in reaching 'normie' friends, as that's the audience I had in mind when writing them. As each article is intended to work on a stand-alone basis, you'll come across some repetition which, I trust, will underscore some of the worst atrocities unleashed under the banner of 'COVID'. You can find and share the individual articles at https://poetseye.substack.com.

Abdiel LeRoy
December 2024

1

PFIZER ADMITS ADOLESCENT VACCINE TRIALS WERE ILLEGAL

Riddle me this. Pfizer tells the FDA it must delay its COVID-vaccine trials in kids because U.S. legislation requires it, but then conducts the trials anyway, causing the paralysis of a 12-year-old girl.

Tragic and bewildering as that sounds, it is what happened in 2020 and 2021, as we now know from court-ordered releases of Pfizer's Biological Product File.

Among more than a thousand documents released so far is *AGREED PEDIATRIC STUDY PLAN,* where Pfizer wrote, "Pfizer and BioNTech propose to request a deferral of the evaluation of the COVID-19 vaccine in individuals ≤15 years of age" (p.8).[1]

This *Study Plan* cites the *Pediatric Research Equity Act of 2003* (21 U.S. Code § 355c) which states, "Pediatric

1. This language is repeated in the document's attachment, *ATTACHMENT A – DEFERRAL REQUEST*

studies should be delayed until additional safety or effectiveness data have been collected" (Section 505B (3) (A)). Thus, Pfizer knew what the legislation required and made it clear that it knew.

The *Study Plan* must have been written after Dec. 18, 2020 because it says Pfizer's and Moderna's COVID jabs had received their initial emergency-use authorizations (EUA) in adults by then, but before May 10, 2021, when Pfizer's EUA was extended down to children between 12 and 15.

Why, then, as chronicled in a *New England Journal of Medicine* (*NEJM*) report, did Pfizer start recruiting children between 12 and 15 for its adolescent clinical trials in October 2020,[2] months before it told the FDA it should wait?

Maddie de Garay

Maddie de Garay was a healthy 12-year-old girl until she received a second Pfizer shot at Cincinnati Children's Hospital on Jan. 20, 2021. About 18 hours after the injection, she started experiencing severe chest pain—it felt like her heart was being pulled out—and a sensation like excruciating electric shocks throughout her neck and spine. Her fingers and toes turned white and were ice

2. "Between October 15, 2020, and January 12, 2021, a total of 2306 adolescents 12 to 15 years of age were screened for inclusion, and 2264 underwent randomization across 29 U.S. sites; 2260 participants received injections, with 1131 receiving BNT162b2 and 1129 receiving placebo."

cold to the touch. The pain in her toes was so intense that she had to walk on her heels. Over the following weeks and months, she became incontinent, paralyzed from the waist down, and could only receive nutrition through a feeding tube.

But Dr. Robert Frenck, director of the Gamble Vaccine Research Center at Cincinnati Children's, and principal investigator for Pfizer's clinical trial in adolescents, told Maddie's parents in a May 17, 2021 phone conversation that the hospital team did not deem her condition to be "research related"—meaning Pfizer's medicine did not cause it—so the family would have to foot Maddie's medical bills themselves.

Then, the following week, on May 27, Frenck appeared as lead author of the *NEJM* article and asserted, based on the trial in which Maddie took part, that Pfizer's vaccine "had a favorable safety and side-effect profile... There were no vaccine-related serious adverse events and few overall severe adverse events" (p.1, p.239).

Here is the bizarre timeline...

- October 2020—Pfizer recruits children aged 12 through 15 for adolescent clinical trials.

- Between Dec. 18, 2020 and May 10, 2021—Pfizer tells FDA that evaluation of COVID-19 vaccine should be deferred in individuals ≤15 years of age to comply with Pediatric Research Equity Act.

- Starting Jan. 20, 2021—12-year-old Maddie de Garay devastated by second Pfizer jab in adolescents trial.

- May 17, 2021—Robert Frenck tells Maddie's parents they're on their own with medical bills.

- May 27, 2021—*NEJM* article asserts that, based on the trial in which Maddie took part, Pfizer "had a favorable safety and side-effect profile... There were no vaccine-related serious adverse events and few overall severe adverse events."

How shall we makes sense of this topsy-turvy course of events? Did the Pfizer author who sought to delay the vaccine's evaluation in adolescents not get the memo that the company was already recruiting the prohibited age group? It's a glaring internal contradiction, but the overall fact remains...

PFIZER UNDERSTOOD IT WAS LEGALLY REQUIRED TO DEFER EVALUATION FOR THE 12-15 AGE GROUP, BUT WENT AHEAD ANYWAY, AND CAUSED TRAGIC HARM BY DOING SO.

2

PFIZER'S PLANDEMIC

You've heard the allegations. That the COVID 'pandemic' was pure fiction, a carefully orchestrated bioterrorism exercise spun out of thin air to usher in totalitarian control by government corporatocracy. Not a pandemic at all, it is said, but a 'plandemic' or 'scamdemic'.

Of course, the powers-that-be ridicule such ideas and their messengers, insisting that—whether by accident or design—a deadly virus erupted upon the world in 2020 and that, to save us from it, we needed global lockdowns, shutdowns, and coerced medical interventions.

But if, as the official narrative contends, COVID took everybody by surprise in 2020, why was Pfizer recruiting clinical-trial investigators for its COVID 'vaccine' in 2018 and 2019?

These questions arise from two PDF files—*Part A* and *Part B*—produced by the FDA as part of its court-ordered release of Pfizer's Biological Product File. These two files comprise the CVs (resumés) of investigators who conducted Pfizer's clinical trials. Some have been duplicated but, broadly speaking, there are about 160 in the pile, of which roughly 130 are fom U.S. investigators, the rest coming from Germany, Turkey, South Africa, Brazil, and Argentina.

As might be expected, most of the CVs are signed between May and August 2020, consistent with the timing of Pfizer's trials, but others are suspiciously premature for the official COVID narrative that warned of a deadly 'pandemic' in early 2020. Three of the CVs are signed in 2018, ten in 2019, and 14 in the first quarter of 2020, together amounting to about 17% of the total. Why was Pfizer recruiting so early?

The zealous recruits include one Robert Wilson Frenck, Jr., MD who covered up the paralysis of 12-year-old Maddie de Garay after she received a second Pfizer shot in adolescent trials he led at Cincinnati Children's Hospital. He signed his CV in February 2019.

Here is a list of the earliest signatories...

- Edward Walsh, Rochester General Hospital, NY, signed Apr. 24, 2018 (Part A, p.49).

- Lisa Cohen, Wake Research Inc., NC, signed May 23, 2018 (Part A, p.112).

- Wayne Harper, M3 Wake Research Inc., NC, signed July 31, 2018 (Part A, p.113).

- Charles Harold Harper, Meridian Clinical Research, NE, signed Jan. 23, 2019 (Part B, p.24).

- Paul Bradley, Meridian Clinical Research, GA, signed Feb. 1, 2019 (Part B, p.17).

- Robert Wilson Frenck, Jr., Gamble Program for Clinical Studies, Cincinnati Children's Hospital Medical Center, signed Feb. 19, 2019 (Part A, p.53).

- Cristiano Zerbini, Centro Paulista de Investigação Clínica, Sao Paulo, Brazil, signed Apr. 17, 2019 (Part A, p.3).

- Douglas Denham, Clinical Trials of Texas, Inc., TX, signed Apr. 15, 2019 (Part A, p.102).

- Sybille Baumann, CRS Clinical Research Services, GmbH, Berlin, signed May 13, 2019 (Part B, p.98).

- Laurence Chu, Benchmark Research, TX, signed May 28, 2019 (Part A, p.101).

- Paul Pickrell, Tekton Research Inc., TX, signed Nov. 19, 2019 (Part A, p.122).

- Aaron N. Hartman, Virginia Research Center, LLC, VA, signed Dec. 2, 2019 (Part A, p.76).

- Helen Lee Stacey, Diablo Clinical Research, CA, signed Dec. 19, 2019 (Part A, p.83).

The early recruitment of these 13 individuals raises the age-old question: What did Pfizer know, and when did it know it?

3

THE DEVIL'S ENZYME

When Internet sleuths discovered that COVID 'vaccines' contain an enzyme called Luciferase, social media was abuzz with speculation. Was this Big Pharma paying tribute to the Father of Lies? Or worse, was it the Mark of the Beast, without which none would be able to buy or sell, as foretold in the Bible's final book, *Revelation*?

What does Pfizer's Biological Product File have to say about this stuff? In *2.4 Nonclinical Overview*, released March 2022, we read that luciferase is extracted from the firefly, pyractomena lucifera. It produces bioluminescence —meaning it makes things glow—so it can be used to track the course of substances injected into the body. We also learn from this document that luciferase was used as a marker for the distribution of components in Pfizer's BNT162b2 'vaccine' product after injection into rats and mice.

Released at the same time was Pfizer's *R&D STUDY*

REPORT No. R-20-0072, which describes experiments on mice "to investigate the biodistribution of luciferase expressed by the LNP-formulated modRNA using bioluminescence measurements."

'LNP' stands for lipid nanoparticles, and 'modRNA' for modified RNA, two controversial components introduced to 'vaccine' technology in the COVID era. This study was conducted in Mainz, Germany between Jan. 14, 2020 and Jan. 23, 2020 (p.8).

So here are three key questions...

- Why was Pfizer testing the technology it would use in its COVID shots in January 2020, almost two months before the World Health Organization declared COVID a "global pandemic" on Mar. 11, 2020?

- Was luciferase used solely as a marker in Pfizer's animal experiments, or was it included in the shots themselves? As discovered by investigative reporter, Emerald Robinson, and reported in her article of Nov. 4, 2021, Moderna lists luciferase as a component of its COVID vaccine in patent US 10,703,789 (p.46, Table 4). What about Pfizer?

- Do COVID shots include technology that can divulge who has, or has not, received them? This would desecrate Medical Confidentiality and Informed Consent, and make a mockery of

> the Hippocratic Oath, but a *Smithsonian* article of December 2019 shows the technology exists. It describes a new microneedle device that "delivers fluorescent nanoparticles beneath the skin." These could then be scanned "and someday allow health providers to archive and access patients' past vaccinations without the muss and fuss of external records." How convenient! The *Smithsonian* article appeared shortly after the U.S. Department of Homeland Security filed Patent 10829770 B2 on Sept. 16, 2019. It describes the use of luciferase —derived in this case from gaussia princeps, a marine crustacean—for "certifying vaccine expression in vivo" (para. 146, p.27).

To date, neither Pfizer nor the FDA has divulged whether luciferase is a component of the Pfizer shot, but Informed Consent requires it let us know.

4

GRANULAR GENOCIDE — PFIZER'S "TINY ASSASSINS"

You may have seen the images. Tiny structures that show up when Pfizer's COVID serums are put under the microscope and that even respond to external stimuli such as electromagnetic fields. You may have also seen images of 'dirty blood', where strange objects appear in samples taken from the injected. It's all very science fiction and drives speculation about what is happening at the 'nano' level—meaning billionths of a meter—in the COVID injections dubbed 'vaccines'.

An alternative term for their novel technology, as used in nature.com, is 'nanomedicine' that uses 'nanotechnology'. As defined by the CDC, nanotechnology means "the manipulation of matter on a near-atomic scale to produce new structures, materials and devices."

Thus, podcasts, video channels, and social media are abuzz with terms like 'nanocircuit', 'nanofiber', 'nanoribbon', 'nanotech', 'nanotube', and 'nanowire'. More exotic variants include 'nanobot', 'nanobox', 'nanocar', 'nanoflower', 'nanopyramid', 'nanosphere', and 'nanostar'.

These terms do not appear in Pfizer's Biological Product File, extracted through protracted lawsuits against the FDA, but 'nanoparticle' appears thousands of times, usually preceded by the word 'lipid', or 'LNP', meaning 'lipid nanoparticle'.

What do Pfizer's documents reveal about these LNPs? First, that they are central to the company's vaccine enterprise. "Vaccine candidates are encapsulated into LNPs," it explains in *2.5 Clinical Overview* (p.19). Also, in a June 2022 article on its website, Pfizer describes LNPs as a "reliable vehicle" to deliver the vaccines' "precious cargo" into human cells.

But what are these LNPs? As usual, there is no low-hanging fruit when it comes to getting disclosure out of Pfizer. Instead, we must tease out the truth from snippets of information prised from its jealous clutches. *2.5 Clinical Overview* tells us, "The LNPs are composed of four different lipids in a defined ratio."

So what are the four? In *R&D STUDY REPORT No. R-20-0072*, also part of Pfizer's Biological Product File, they are listed as 'amino-lipid' ALC-0315; 'PEG-lipid' ALC-0159; 'phospholipid' DSPC (distearoyl-phosphocholine); and cholesterol (p.4 and p.12).

These terms mean little-to-nothing to the lay person, perhaps by design, but medical literature tells us the overall purpose of these LNPs in vaccines is to provide a protective structure to deliver genetic material into human cells—a process called 'transfection'—without interference from the pesky immune system.

But is this technology safe? According to another nature.com article of Aug. 10, 2021, it hasn't even been proven safe in animals, let alone humans. "In vivo application of lipid nanoparticles has been reported to induce liver and lung injuries in rodents," the analysis warns (p.10).

Pfizer's documents admit the potential harms of LNPs in rodents too. For example, as reported in *2.4 Nonclinical Overview,* LNPs accumulate in rats' livers following injection, and "Fibrinogen was higher in the vaccine-administered group (up to 3.1x controls)." This signals an increased risk of blood clots.

Pfizer's closest rival, Moderna, also highlighted the potential dangers of LNPs in a corporate prospectus it submitted to the Securities and Exchange Commission (SEC) in 2018. "Most of our investigational medicines are formulated and administered in an LNP which may lead to systemic side effects related to the components of the LNP which may not have ever been tested in humans. While we have continued to optimize our LNPs, there can be no assurance that our LNPs will not have undesired effects."

We are also alerted to the specific dangers of the ALC-0315 particle in a product insert from Cayman Chemical, a biochemical manufacturer based in Ann Arbor, MI. It describes ALC-0315 as a cationic lipid "used in the development of LNPs for the delivery of mRNA-based vaccines."

Warnings follow: "THIS PRODUCT IS FOR RESEARCH ONLY—NOT FOR HUMAN OR VETERINARY DIAGNOSTIC OR THERAPEUTIC USE… This material should be considered hazardous until further information becomes available. Do not ingest, inhale, get in eyes, on skin, or on clothing. Wash thoroughly after handling" (emphasis included).

So it's OK to inject this into people but not to inhale or ingest it? And it's not considered safe for man or beast? And what of the term, 'cationic'? This means that a particle hosts a positive electronic charge which, according to ThermoFisher Scientific, allows for fusion with a negatively charged cell membrane.

Cationic LNPs are "very, very toxic," according to cell biologist, Dr. Vanessa Schmidt-Kruger, in an August 2021 article published by Weston A. Price Foundation. "Cationic lipids can interact with DNA and create strand breaks, and also interact with negatively charged lipids in the membrane of the mitochondria—the cellular powerhouses that produce energy. This can set in motion a series of toxic reactions: destruction of the mitochondrial membrane, formation of free radicals that damage the cell, disruption of ion balance, loss of cellular function, and DNA damage. Ultimately, the cell will either self-destruct or turn into a cancer cell." A few months later, in December 2021, an article in *iScience* warned, "The cationic lipid component of the lipid carriers is often inflammatory."

And what of ALC-0159, the next LNP in the list? Is that any safer than its cationic cousin? This is the 'PEG-lipid', where 'PEG' stands for polyethylene glycol. Here, Cayman Chemical has another product insert issuing the exact same warnings.

PEG LNPs "are a way you get something everywhere, the brain, the testicles, the ovaries, the unborn child, the unborn child's brain, etc.," said Canadian doctor, Mark Trozzi, in an interview with Odessa Orlewicz. "That's known. That's what that kind of gun does when you fire it." Meanwhile, medical literature warns that PEG has a track record of causing "severe allergic symptoms with occasionally fatal anaphylaxis." In short,...

PFIZER'S COVID PRODUCT CONTAINS PARTICLES KNOWN TO PROMOTE BLOOD CLOTS, CANCER, AND DEATH.

Furthermore, if Pfizer's serum contains graphene nanoparticles—described in *The Exposé* as "tiny assassins" and "silent destroyers"—then the toxicity concerns become more pressing still. According to a 2016 article in *Particle and Fibre Toxicology*, graphene-family nanoparticles exhibit several mechanisms of toxicity, including "physical destruction, oxidative stress, DNA damage, inflammatory response, apoptosis, autophagy, and necrosis."

I have found just one occurrence of 'graphene' in the FDA's document releases so far. Though deeply embedded in impenetrable scientific jargon, it demonstrates that graphene is used in the vaccine manufacturing process (p.7).

LNP Sources

So where does Pfizer get its LNPs? The aforementioned *R&D Study Report* mentions several times that each of the four types is licensed from Acuitas Therapeutics in British Columbia, Canada. According to Acuitas' website, the company has "synthesized over 500 novel cationic lipids" and "shown that the ionizable cationic lipid component critically determines the potency of LNP therapeutics."

So Acuitas has a potent product, but is it a safe one? A December 2021 article in *iScience* reported that Acuitas' LNPs, used in messenger-RNA (mRNA) vaccine studies, caused "massive local inflammation" in mice.

Another document in Pfizer's Biological Product File, *INVESTIGATION OF THE BIOTRANSFORMATION OF ALC-0159 AND ALC-0315 IN VITRO AND IN VIVO IN RATS,* states that Alabama-based Avanti Polar Lipids Inc. is the source of LNPs (p.4). According to Avanti's website, it was acquired in 2020 by pharmaceutical company, Croda International Plc, by which "we were collectively able to supply the lipid components needed for clinical trials and the commercial launch of the Covid-19 vaccine." Meanwhile, LNPs are so lucrative for pharma companies in general that they are squabbling over the spoils through patent litigation.

Self-Assembly?

Another concerning prospect with injected nanoparticles is self-assembly. Bizarre as that sounds, self-assembling nanoparticles are a technology explicitly stated in one of Moderna's patents for its COVID-19 Spikevax serum. The patent, US 10703789, applies to "self-assembled" and "fully programmable" nanoparticles (para. 219).

But the technology can be traced back further to 2013 in another patent for "inventive vaccine nanocarriers," US 9,539,210 B2, filed by Massachusetts Institute of Technology and others. In some embodiments, "the nanocarrier is formed by self-assembly… In some embodiments, the nanocarrier is a microparticle, nanoparticle, or picoparticle. In some embodiments, the microparticle, nanoparticle, or picoparticle is self-assembled."

This is where nanotechnology become indistinguishable from weaponry. "In some embodiments," the patent continues, "the small molecule is a toxin. In some embodiments, the toxin is from a chemical weapon, an agent of biowarfare, or a hazardous environmental agent."

And it appears this potential for weaponization has been embraced by the U.S. military. For example, in a 2018 presentation at West Point Military Academy, neuroscientist Dr. James Giordano boasted, "I can create small robotic units, controllable robotic units at the nanoscale, and that these too can be aerosolized to create a nanoswarm, a biopenetrable material that you cannot see, that can penetrate all but the most robust biochemical filters, that are able to integrate themselves through a variety of membranes, mucus membranes and wherever—mouth, nose, ears, eyes—can be then uptaken into the vascular system to create clumping, can affect the vascular system of the brain or can directly diffuse into the brain space, and these can be weaponized. And it can be done in such a level that their presence is almost impossible to detect and, as such, the attribution becomes exceedingly difficult to demonstrate."

Even more recently, at a Mar. 21, 2023 seminar of the Autonomous Robotics Research Center, telecommunications professor Ian Akyildiz described mRNA in COVID vaccines as "nano-scale machines" that are "programmed, and they're injected" (13:40).

Nanoparticles in General

Scientists have long known the dangers of nanoparticles in general. For example, a 2005 paper titled *Nanotoxicology: an emerging discipline from studies of ultrafine particles* warned that, once in the bloodstream, nanoparticles can distribute throughout the body, finding their way to the liver, heart, kidney, spleen, and bone marrow.

And, in a 2014 book titled *Nanomaterials for Environmental Protections*, the authors warn, "With the decrease in size, there is an increase in the inherent toxicity of nanoparticles," and that "Prolonged exposure to nanoparticles can have an adverse effect on human health and the environment."

Nanoparticles can also damage DNA and cause cellular death, according to the book. They "enter the body by inhalation, injection into the bloodstream, and passage through the skin. They also have the potential to penetrate the blood–brain barrier due to their small size. Nanoparticles can interact with proteins and enzymes, alter gene expression, and thus affect the biological behavior at the organ, tissue, cellular, subcellular, and protein levels."

Since then, as reported in *NewScientist* in 2015, "Carbon nanotubes have turned up in the lungs of children living in Paris–the first time they have been detected in humans." Researchers at the University of Paris-Saclay, France, "studied fluid from the airways of 64 asthmatic children, and discovered carbon nanotubes in all of the samples."

Then there are the harms to reproductive tissues, as chronicled in a 2018 study titled *Potential adverse effects of nanoparticles on the reproductive system*. Along with toxic effects on the brain, liver and kidney, nanoparticles can accumulate in, and damage, ovaries, the uterus, and testes, and adversely affect sperm quality, quantity, and motility. Nanoparticles can also affect the development of offspring, according to the paper.

So where is the Informed Consent for these microscopic objects of momentous import? When it comes to Pfizer's nanoparticles, the devil really *is* in the details!

5

DR. ROBERT FRENCK: COVID'S UNSUNG VILLAIN

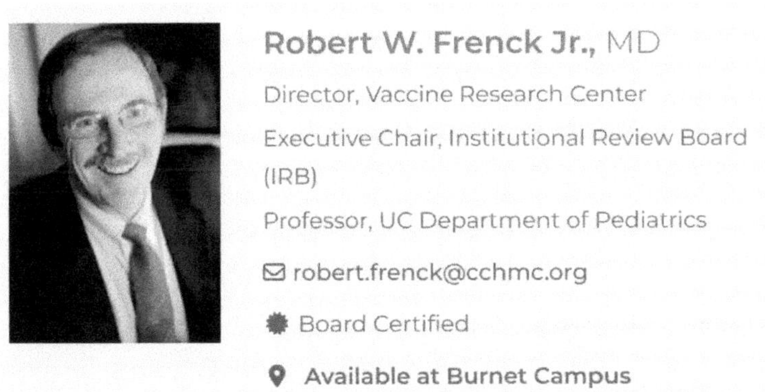

It must be gratifying for Dr. Robert Frenck to sit atop a major vaccine research center in Cincinnati and do the godly work of Pfizer. "I'm an acknowledged authority in infectious diseases," he crows in his bio, "and have authored more than 125 articles and book chapters."

And we're all very impressed. Frenck may not be a

household name like Fauci or Gates, Walensky or Woodcock, or any of the other prominent actors in the COVID era, but his exploits are no less noteworthy. As director of the Gamble Vaccine Research Center at Cincinnati Children's Hospital, he oversaw Pfizer's clinical trials for adolescents aged 12 through 15, which would have a momentous impact on official policy in the following months and years.

Illegal Trials

These trials were illegal, according to Pfizer's own understanding of U.S. legislation. In *AGREED PEDIATRIC STUDY PLAN*, part of Pfizer's Biological Product File extracted from the FDA through legal process, Pfizer wrote, "Pfizer and BioNTech propose to request a deferral of the evaluation of the COVID-19 vaccine in individuals ≤15 years of age" (p.8).

To support this request, Pfizer cited the Pediatric Research Equity Act of 2003 (21 U.S. Code § 355c) which states, "Pediatric studies should be delayed until additional safety or effectiveness data have been collected" (Section 505B (3)(A)). Thus, Pfizer knew what the legislation required and made it clear that it knew.

The *Study Plan* must have been written after Dec. 18, 2020 because it mentions that both Pfizer's and Moderna's COVID jabs had received their initial 'emergency-use authorizations' (EUA) in adults. These occurred on Dec. 11, 2020 and Dec. 18, 2020, respectively. And it must have preceded the FDA's EUA extension for Pfizer down to 12-year-olds on May 10, 2021.

Why, then, as chronicled in a *New England Journal of Medicine* (*NEJM*) article, did Pfizer begin recruiting 12- to 15-year-old children for its adolescent clinical trials in October 2020 (p.5), months before Pfizer told the FDA it should wait to comply with legal requirements?

Should we dwell on this, though? Perhaps Frenck was not familiar with the applicable legislation, and maybe he was not briefed on Pfizer's communications with the FDA as he conducted these trials. Besides, why worry about mere illegality when you've got a world to save and a miraculous serum to dispense?

Frenck must have been eager for the role as, with remarkable foresight, he signed up to be a clinical investigator for Pfizer on Feb. 19, 2019, more than a year before the World Health Organization declared a global COVID 'pandemic' on Mar. 11, 2020.

Current Position at Study Site: *current affiliation as noted in box 3 of the Form FDA 1572 or ICH GCP Attestation*

Start Date	Title	Institution or Company	State/Province & Country
2006- Present	Professor of Pediatrics	Cincinnati Children's Hospital Medical Center	OH, USA

Previous Relevant Positions Including Academic Appointments: *provide previous 4 relevant positions if applicable*

Start and End Dates	Title	Institution or Company	Country
2004-2006	Professor of Pediatrics	University of California at Los Angles	USA
1997-Present	Associate Professor of Pediatrics	Uniformed Services, University of Health and Science, MD	USA
1994-1997	Associate Professor of Pediatrics	Eastern Virginia Medical School, VA	USA

Brief Summary of Relevant Clinical Research Experience: *Enter "None" if no previous clinical research experience*

Clinical Studies in the Division of Infectious Diseases at CCHMC conducts research on the prevention, diagnosis, and management of infections in subjects of all ages. PI and sub-I on numerous industry, government and PI initiated studies. PI on many studies both in military & civilian, numerous publications, academic & administrative committees, scientific review/consult & professional organizations.

Signature: *This CV is to be signed and dated by the investigator to whom the CV applies. If the investigator refuses to sign, indicate "Refusal to Sign" and date of refusal in the Signature Date box.*	Signature Date: (dd-Mmm-yyyy)
[signature]	19 Feb 2019

I will update and resubmit my abbreviated CV if there are changes and particularly if there is any change in status which would adversely affect the assessment of my suitability to conduct/participate in clinical studies.

Frenck was one of 13 investigators who signed their CV (resumé) before the end of 2019, as we now know from documents Part A and Part B, also part of Pfizer's Biological Product File. Frenck's CV is in Part A, p.53.

Of course, we could give Frenck another pass on this too. Perhaps it was mere coincidence that he and the other investigators just happened to be in the right place at the right time when a new and terrifying disease showed up.

Maddie de Garay

But the harms to children on Frenck's watch are not so easily explained. Maddie de Garay was one of those children. On Jan. 20, 2021, at the age of 12, she received a second dose of Pfizer's 'BNT162b2' concoction in Frenck's two-dose trial for adolescents at Cincinnati Children's Hospital. About 18 hours later, she developed severe nerve pain, a feeling like electric shocks going down her neck and spine, excruciating abdominal pain, and severe chest pain that felt like her heart was being pulled out. Her vaccine arm swelled up and became numb. Her fingers and toes turned white, and were ice cold to the touch. The pain in her toes was so bad that she had to walk on her heels.

Over the following months, Maddie's condition worsened, including food regurgitation and vomiting, until she was unable to swallow any food or liquids, and had to resort to a feeding tube. The pain throughout her body persisted, especially in her abdomen, which became distended. She experienced fainting spells which developed into seizures, sometimes 10 a day.

Prior to injection, Maddie had never menstruated, but on Feb. 5, 2021, she started to discharge brown fluid, which came out in chunks over the following month. Painful cysts developed on her vagina and then her head. Erratic blood pressure and heart rate were also among the symptoms, along with tinnitus, vision problems, headaches, dizziness, and memory loss. Finally, she lost feeling from the waist down, which led to paralysis and incontinence.

International Protections

The *Nuremberg Code* of 1947, which applies to experimental medicine, states, "During the course of the experiment the scientist in charge must be prepared to terminate the experiment at any stage, if he has probable cause to believe, in the exercise of the good faith, superior skill and careful judgment required of him, that a continuation of the experiment is likely to result in injury, disability, or death to the experimental subject" (Para. 10).

But Frenck did not terminate the experiment. In his lead-authored article describing the trial in which Maddie participated, which appeared in *The New England Journal of Medicine* (*NEJM*) on May 27, 2021, we learn that the trial ran until its data cut-off point of Mar. 13, 2021 (p.2), almost two months after Maddie got her second Pfizer shot on Jan. 20, 2021. Worse yet, Frenck asserted Pfizer's vaccine "had a favorable safety and side-effect profile... there were no vaccine-related serious adverse events and few overall severe adverse events" (p.1).

Yet Frenck added yet more insult to Maddie's injuries when, in a May 17, 2021 phone call with Maddie's parents, Stephanie and Patrick, he said Pfizer would not cover the staggering medical bills Maddie had run up at Cincinnati Children's in trying to cope with her debilitation. "The doctors that have seen her so far have not found something where they thought it was research related," he said, meaning his team deemed Maddie's injuries unattributable to the clinical trial.

Again, he was desecrating international law. As stated in the Declaration of Helsinki—Ethical Principles for Medical Research Involving Human Subjects, "Appropriate compensation and treatment for subjects who are harmed as a result of participating in research must be ensured" (Para. 15).

Frenck's Whitewashing Frenzy

In Pfizer's first *Periodic Safety Update Report* (*PSUR #1*) to the European Medicines Agency (EMA), released in early 2023, Maddie's designation of 'Abdominal pain' is listed among 17 adverse events for her age group in clinical trials alone (p.228). Distributed among 14 children, the events are: "Depression (4), Suicidal ideation (3), Appendicitis (2), Abdominal pain, Anal abscess, Anxiety, Constipation, Conversion disorder, Femur fracture and Focal peritonitis (1 each)."

The report then claims, "All events were assessed as unrelated to BNT162b2 or blinded therapy" (p.228). This raises the question: if Frenck could describe Maddie's paralysis as 'abdominal pain' and rule that it was unrelated to Pfizer's medicine, what were his omissions and oversights when it came to the 13 other injured children and the 16 other adverse events?

Frenck's role in facilitating Pfizer's encroachments into childhood, and even into the cradle, should not be underestimated. As he boasted in the *NEJM* article, Pfizer's EUA was extended to 12-year-olds "on the basis of data presented in this report." This opened the door for EUA extensions for Pfizer to five-year-olds in October 2021 and to six-month-olds in June 2022.

Frenck's fraud doesn't stop there, though. The article states that the study recorded unsolicited adverse events reported by trial participants until six months after dose two (p.3), but that is a chronological impossibility given the study's data cut-off date of Mar. 13, 2021 (p.2).

Another Bogus Trial

Yet Pfizer must have been pleased with Frenck's performance because he led another study at Cincinnati Children's Hospital from February 2021 to July 2021, this time into Pfizer's 'lot consistency' (Protocol C4591017), including a safety comparison across different manufacturing lots of BNT162b2.

But the study's structure alone set the stage for another whitewash. To begin with, it assessed only four manufacturing lots, three from the U.S. and one from Europe. Compare that with the 4,756 Pfizer lot numbers listed at howbad.info, a searchable independent database that tallies injuries per lot from various manufacturers of COVID 'vaccines'. Or compare Frenck's paltry four lots with the 52 batch numbers deployed in Denmark alone, or with the 19 lot numbers associated with the highest numbers of adverse events according to *PSUR #1*.

Meanwhile, huge inconsistencies have been observed in the toxicity and lethality of Pfizer's COVID jabs, depending on their batch numbers, but those numbers cannot be correlated with Frenck's lame study which refers to its test lots only as 'US Lot 1', 'US Lot 2', 'US Lot 3', and 'EU Lot'.

Furthermore, the evaluation ran only until one month after Dose 2 (or one month after Dose 3 in 62 participants who got a 'booster' shot), severely curtailing its scope for recording adverse events. Even so, among 1,574 participants, two 'serious adverse events' (SAE) were noted. One involved "exposure during pregnancy followed by an SAE of spontaneous abortion," and the other experienced status-migrainosus. The investigators determined, however, that "neither were related to the study vaccine." The study also logged eight cases of lymphadenopathy (swelling of the lymph nodes) and one case each of dermatitis and angioedema.

Yet the paper glibly concludes, "Safety profiles across all vaccine groups were similar with no safety concerns identified in both the primary and booster study. Vaccines in all arms of the study were well-tolerated in both the primary and booster study. The safety profile was consistent with previous studies."

In Closing...

I reached out to Dr. Frenck several times for comment, both by phone and email, but he failed to respond, leaving me to draw my own conclusions—that his allegiance lies not with medicine but with Molech, and that his accursed name must not be excluded from the forthcoming measures of Justice against murderers of this age. He has lied from start to finish, played fast and loose with lives and legislation, and repeatedly desecrated the Hippocratic Oath along the way. That he is still at large, let alone practising, is an indictment of our medical and legal systems combined. I give the last word to my friend JP who added his own comment after reading my assessment of Frenck...

> What a DISGUSTING individual!
> He carried out ILLEGAL tests on children.
> He LIED about results.
> He SEVERELY injured several children.
> He REFUSED to admit responsibility.
> He PROMOTED further use of vaccines.
> He BOASTS about being "an acknowledged authority."
> He should be INJECTED with the batch he gave to young Maddie.

After 6 months of (hopefully) excruciating pain, he should be HUNG.

And as my friend added:

Then he should be dug up, and hung a second time.

Then he should be drawn and quartered, and then hung a third time.

6

SECOND-HAND VACCINATION

You will often hear the word 'shedding' or 'transmission' when people talk about Pfizer's COVID 'vaccine'. It suggests that components of the shot, along with components that the injected also produce in their own bodies, are being spread from one body to another. The term also suggests that the unvaccinated are getting Pfizer's medicine, whether they want it or not. But what does Pfizer's Biological Product File, extracted by legal process from the FDA, have to say about this?

Sullied Sperm

Pfizer's *Participant information leaflet,* dated July 2020, tells clinical-trial participants, "Men may not donate sperm until 60 days after the last vaccination" (p.18, p.130). So what is in the sperm of injected men that can harm their sexual partners or potential offspring or both?

Perhaps clinical-trial participant 12314384 would know. As recorded in *Listing of Adverse Events*, another document in Pfizer's file, he experienced "Ejaculation disorder/ brownish ejaculation" in November 2020, within two months of receiving a second Pfizer dose in the company's main C4591001 clinical trial (p.3,350). Of course, the trial investigator determined this affliction was not 'Vax Rel'.

16.2.7.4.1 Listing of Adverse Events – All Subjects ≥16 Years of Age

Age Group (Years)/ Subject	System Organ Class	Preferred Term/ AE Investigator Text	Dose No.	Onset Date	Rel Day[a]/ Dur (Days)[b]	Toxicity Grade	Vax Rel[c]	Cause of AE	Action: Investigational Vaccine Dose/ Subject	Outcome (End Date)	SAE/Imm AE (Yes/No)
>55/ C4591001 1231 12314384	REPRO	Ejaculation disorder/ brownish ejaculation	2	13NOV2020	58/3	1	No	O	NA	R (15NOV2020)	N/N

That vaccine components make their way from the injection site to vital organs of the body, including reproductive organs, we know from Pfizer's *Tissue Distribution Study*, conducted on rats. It observed rapid accumulation of 'lipid nanoparticles' (LNP) in the testes and uterus through to 48 hours post-injection, at which point the data gathering was stopped (p.24).

Results expressed as total lipid concentration (µg l

Sample	Total Lipid Concentration (µg lipid equiv/g (or mL))						
	0.25 min	1 h	2 h	4 h	8 h	24 h	48 h
Small intestine	0.030	0.221	0.476	0.879	1.279	1.302	1.472
Spinal cord	0.043	0.097	0.169	0.250	0.106	0.085	0.112
Spleen	0.334	2.471	7.734	10.296	22.091	20.080	23.353
Stomach	0.017	0.065	0.115	0.144	0.268	0.152	0.215
Testes (males)	0.031	0.042	0.079	0.129	0.146	0.304	0.320
Thymus	0.088	0.243	0.340	0.335	0.196	0.207	0.331
Thyroid	0.155	0.536	0.842	0.851	0.544	0.578	1.000
Uterus (females)	0.043	0.203	0.305	0.140	0.287	0.289	0.456

More precautions for male trial subjects are set out in Pfizer's *dose-finding study*. In addition to refraining from sperm donation, in this case only for "at least 28 days after the last dose of study intervention," participants are told either to abstain from intercourse "with a female of childbearing potential" or to use a condom (Appendix 4, p.140).

But even that may not be enough because, in addition to male condom use, "a highly effective method of contraception may be considered" in the men's partners if they are of child-bearing potential. The same warning was not issued for sexual partners outside of childbearing age, suggesting that the precautions were mostly about shielding potential offspring.

Eggs Defiled

The *Clinical Trial Protocol* also specifies female participants "of childbearing age may not donate eggs until 60 days after the last vaccination." They must also test negative for pregnancy at the start of the trial and for 60 days after receiving the last immunization. The criteria also excluded women who were breastfeeding, or planned to breastfeed, until at least 90 days after the last immunization.

Tragedies Transplacental and Transmammary

Yet, for all the measures stipulated in Pfizer's trials, the public rollout of its COVID product was recklessly cavalier. In its *Cumulative Analysis* report, Pfizer records 26 spontaneous abortions and one neonatal death among 28 known outcomes for prenatal children when their mothers had received Pfizer's serum. There was but one known "normal outcome" during the reporting period (p.12).[1]

This report was based on adverse-event notices Pfizer received from 63 countries starting in December 2020, when regulatory authorizations began, and the end of February 2021. The numbers were gleaned from voluntary reports alone so that, as the document states, "the magnitude of underreporting is unknown."

Meanwhile, Pfizer gleaned early clues about possible harms to infants breastfeeding from vaccinated mothers, including reports of suppressed lactation and breastmilk discoloration. Shortly after, reports of breastfeeding infant deaths started to appear in the Vaccine Adverse Events Reporting System (VAERS), a database jointly managed by the FDA and CDC.

The earliest reports in VAERS include...

- A six-week-old boy who died on July 17, 2021 "from clots in his severely inflamed arteries," as

1. This calculation is derived from the following text in Pfizer's document: "Pregnancy outcomes for the 270 pregnancies were reported as spontaneous abortion (23), outcome pending (5), premature birth with neonatal death, spontaneous abortion with intrauterine death (2 each), spontaneous abortion with neonatal death, and normal outcome (1 each). No outcome was provided for 238 pregnancies (note that 2 different outcomes were reported for each twin, and both were counted)."

reported to VAERS by his 36-year-old mother. "I had been breastfeeding my 6 week old baby at the time that I received the first Pfizer vaccine... I am curious if the spike protein could have gone through the breast milk and caused an inflammatory response in my child" (VAERS ID: 1532154).

- A five-month-old boy who died soon after his mother got a second Pfizer dose on March 17, 2021. The next day, he "developed a rash and within 24 hours was inconsolable, refusing to eat, and developed a fever. Patient brought baby to local ER where assessments were performed, blood analysis revealed elevated liver enzymes. Infant was hospitalized but continued to decline and passed away. Diagnosis of TTP. No known allergies. No new exposures aside from the mother's vaccination the previous day" (VAERS ID: 1166062).

- A one-year-old boy who went into intense febrile seizures on Feb. 19, 2021 after "vaccine exposure via breast milk." His mother had received a first Pfizer dose four days earlier (VAERS ID: 1161763).

As we have seen, harmful serum components can be passed from male to female during intercourse. They can also be passed from mother to child, both in the womb and at the breast. Alarming as all that sounds, the transmissibility doesn't stop there, as even breath and touch are vectors of transmission. In the *dose-finding study*, Pfizer specifies that an 'exposure during pregnancy' (EDP) occurs if "A female family member or healthcare provider reports that she is pregnant after having been exposed to the study intervention by inhalation or skin contact." Even a man exposed to the vaccine by inhalation or skin contact can cause an EDP to his female partner, the document adds.

Second-hand vaccination, then, appears at least as transmissible as second-hand smoking or as any supposed virus. Through its novel COVID concoction, Pfizer has ushered in a brave new medical world that makes a mockery of Informed Consent.

7

WARP-SPEED AND PHARMAGEDDON

Recall those breathless days of 2020 when Donald Trump hailed 'Operation Warp Speed'? "The single greatest mobilization in U.S. history," he called it in a Nov. 13, 2020 speech, "pioneering, developing, and manufacturing therapies and vaccines in record time. Numbers like nobody has seen before."

Our cultural lore warns about rushing things, though, doesn't it—haste making waste, *The Hare and the Tortoise*, and so on? Yet Trump boasted, "No medical breakthrough of this scope and magnitude has ever been achieved this rapidly, this quickly."

But at what cost, Mr. Trump? What corners were cut in bringing to market Pfizer's 'vaccine' by emergency-use authorization, even before the year was out, on Dec. 11, 2020? And how often did the alleged need for speed circumvent customary checks and balances in drug development, let alone a drug using a new technology with no track record?

For example, in a European Parliament hearing of Oct. 11, 2022, MEP Rob Roos asked Pfizer executive, Janine Small, “Was the Pfizer COVID vaccine tested on stopping the transmission of the virus before it entered the market?”

“No,” Small replied with a laugh. “These, um, you know, we had to really move at the speed of science to really understand what is taking place in the market.”

This “speed-of-science” argument is in stark contrast to the glacial pace at which the FDA intended to release Pfizer’s Biological Product File. On Aug. 23, 2021, the agency granted formal licensure to Pfizer’s serum for individuals aged 16 and over. Henceforth, it was no longer in emergency-use status but garlanded with the FDA’s endorsement as safe and effective. This brought into play federal regulations that require the FDA to make safety and effectiveness data “immediately available for public disclosure” after a vaccine license is issued (21 C.F.R. § 601.51).

The FDA failed to do so, then refused to do so, but on Sept. 16, 2021, nonprofit group Public Health and Medical Professionals for Transparency (PHMPT) filed suit against the FDA in the Northern District of Texas. At first, the FDA proposed to produce Pfizer’s papers at a paltry 500 pages a month, which would have stretched the release over several decades, but on Jan. 6, 2022, District Judge Mark T. Pittman ruled the FDA must produce at least 55,000 pages per month.

The papers released so far show how aggressively Pfizer cut corners in the name of urgency and emergency. In its *Dose-Finding Study*, we see it changed the protocols for its human vaccine trials seven times between May 13, 2020 and Oct. 6, 2020 (pages 2-9). Were these changes enhancing safety monitoring, or eroding it?

In *Protocol amendment* 2 of the document, dated May 27, 2020, Pfizer "Removed hemoglobin change-from-baseline abnormalities from the laboratory abnormality grading scale as abnormalities should be graded based upon absolute values." Pfizer was effectively saying it could ignore swings in hemoglobin levels among its injected subjects, no matter how dramatic, provided they remained within a range.

How important is hemoglobin (or haemoglobin)? According to World Health Organization guidance for blood donors, "Haemoglobin (Hb) is a protein found in the red blood cells that carries oxygen in your body and gives blood its red colour." In short, it's the stuff of life.

Bear in mind too that 'Paroxysmal nocturnal haemoglobinuria' is listed among 'Adverse Events of Special Interest' in the appendix of Pfizer's *Cumulative Analysis* report. According to Wikipedia, this condition is "a rare, acquired, life-threatening disease of the blood characterized by destruction of red blood cells by the complement system, a part of the body's innate immune system."

In other words, haemoglobinuria is an autoimmune disease that turns the body's immune system against its own red blood cells. As the Bible reminds us, "the life is in the blood" (Leviticus 17:11), but Pfizer gave itself an out with this core metric.

We also learn from the *Dose Finding Study* that, at this point, Pfizer had five 'vaccine candidates'. They were labelled BNT162a1, BNT162b1, BNT162b2, BNT162b3, and BNT162c2, but by *Protocol amendment 5*, dated Jul. 24, 2020, Pfizer had put all its chips on the BNT162b2 candidate.

Adolescent Trials

Then in *Amendment 7*, dated Oct. 6, 2020, Pfizer committed one of its gravest breaches of medical ethics yet—reducing the lower age range of its clinical trials "to include adolescents 12 to 15 years of age."

And sure enough, Pfizer began recruiting 12-15-year-olds as trial subjects just nine days later, on Oct. 15, 2020, as chronicled in a *New England Journal of Medicine* (*NEJM*) article (p.243) of May 2021. "Between October 15, 2020, and January 12, 2021," the article reports, "a total of 2306 adolescents 12 to 15 years of age were screened for inclusion."

Yet this move was in spectacular contradiction to its own later request to the FDA—which appears in *AGREED PEDIATRIC STUDY PLAN*—for "a deferral of the evaluation of the COVID-19 vaccine in individuals ≤15 years of age." This request cited the *Pediatric Research Equity Act of 2003* (21 U.S. Code § 355c) which states, "Pediatric studies should be delayed until additional safety or effectiveness data have been collected."

The *NEJM* paper was lead authored by Dr. Robert Frenck at Cincinnati Children's Hospital, Pfizer's principal investigator for these trials. It claimed Pfizer's vaccine "had a favorable safety and side-effect profile... there were no vaccine-related serious adverse events and few overall severe adverse events."

This was a lie, and Frenck knew it. One of the trial participants at this hospital was Maddie de Garay. Previously a healthy 12-year-old girl, she was paralyzed from the waist down after she received a second Pfizer shot on Jan. 20, 2021. She ended up in a wheelchair, incontinent, and needed a feeding tube to receive nutrition. Yet Frenck not only silenced her agony in his report but told the family they would have to cover Maddie's staggering medical bills themselves!

Lot-Consistency Trials

In another document from Pfizer's Biological Product File, titled *2.5 Clinical Overview*, Pfizer lists eight more clinical studies planned for 2021 (p.24). One is titled 'Lot consistency', with protocol number C4591017, and Frenck led this one too at Cincinnati Children's.

Honest investigation of lot consistency is certainly a crying need for those injured by Pfizer's jab, given the huge inconsistencies in toxicity and lethality observed, but Pfizer's study, which ran from February to July 2021, was a joke. Only four manufacturing lots were assessed, three in the U.S. and one from Europe, compared to the 4,756 Pfizer lot numbers listed at howbad.info, a searchable independent database that tallies injuries per lot from various manufacturers. Denmark alone deployed 52 different BNT162b2 batch numbers, and Pfizer's first *Periodic Safety Update Report to the European Union* (*PSUR #1*), obtained by FOIA request in January 2023, listed 19 lot numbers associated with the highest numbers of adverse events.

The most frequently reported lot numbers in case reports (≥2000 cases) are listed in Table 9 below.

Table 9. Most Frequently Reported Lot Numbers

Lot Number	Number of Cases
EL1484	16077
EJ6797	11168
EK9788	10139
EM0477	9214
EJ6136	7034
EJ6134	7029
EJ6795	7010
EJ6796	4942
EJ6788	4421
EL0725	3870
ER1741	3692
EJ6789	3136
EJ6790	2992
ER1749	2762
EP9598	2750
EL1491	2621
EJ3002	2602
EP9605	2461
EK1768	2157

CONFIDENTIAL
Page 56

So Pfizer's lot-consistency study was built on wobbly foundations from the start. Even so, among 1,574 participants, it recorded two 'serious adverse events' (SAE). One involved "exposure during pregnancy followed by an SAE of spontaneous abortion," and the other experienced status-migrainosus. Frenck determined, of course, that "neither were related to the study vaccine." The study also logged eight cases of lymphadenopathy (swelling of the lymph nodes).

Furthermore, the investigation only ran until one month after Dose 2, or one month after Dose 3 in the 62 participants who got a 'booster' shot, yet Frenck glibly concluded, "Safety profiles across all vaccine groups were similar with no safety concerns identified in both the primary and booster study. Vaccines in all arms of the study were well-tolerated in both the primary and booster study. The safety profile was consistent with previous studies."

So, FDA, how many times does Pfizer get to drop the ball before you drop the hammer? And when does complacency become criminality? In its reckless haste to get its product to market, Pfizer managed to evade true oversight of its trials while the FDA looked the other way, and any inconvenient task that slowed the race to profit was casually cast aside in the name of urgency. Pfizer went through the motions for appearances' sake, but it was all theater and puppetry, a subterfuge to keep the public in the dark. So much for Informed Consent!

8

PFIZER'S SUBTLE MURDERS: COVER-UPS IN CLINICAL TRIALS

IT'S A GRIM READ...

Among the Pfizer papers extracted from the FDA through legal action, several thousand pages bear witness to horrors suffered by clinical-trial participants in 2020 and early 2021, as Pfizer rushed to unleash its COVID 'vaccine' upon the world.

We don't know their names, only numbers, but their individual stories distill the agony of multitudes. Row upon row, their symptoms cry out in a document titled *16.2.7.4.1 Listing of Adverse Events*, part of the FDA's July 2022 release from Pfizer's Biological Product File.

Among the recorded conditions that befell trial participants after they received Pfizer's BNT162b2 injection are: heart disorders, including pericarditis and tachycardia; kidney failure; liver failure; abnormal cell development and cancer; neurological conditions;

spontaneous abortion; gynecological disorders including vaginal infection, vaginal discharge, and uterine bleeding; brain injuries; psychological maladies, such as psychosis; and death.

You have likely heard Big Pharma's protestations that, just because someone fell ill or died *after* they received its medicine, doesn't mean they got sick or died *from* the medicine, the old "correlation-doesn't-mean-causation" ploy. This bias is evident in Pfizer's *Listing of Adverse Events* document, where each injured trial participant is recorded in a row of a table. From page 77, the table's eighth column is titled 'Vax Rel', where every individual gets a 'Yes' or 'No' in the corresponding cell.

The 'Yes' entries are overwhelmingly applied to milder conditions, while the deadlier outcomes usually get a 'No'. Are these entries true? Or do they reflect a bias among the trial investigators on Pfizer's payroll?

This question is answered in another bundle of documents released by the FDA in July 2022, where post-vaccination symptoms are described in open-ended text fields. It doesn't have a heading, so I'll call it *Narratives*. Spanning 3,611 pages, it lists for each trial participant, "Reason(s) for Narrative" and whether they got Pfizer's BNT162b2 or a placebo.

The very first case is a 56-year-old white female who did get Pfizer's medicine and "died because of cardiac arrest on 21 Oct 2020, 62 days after receiving Dose 2" (p.6). Tests also showed brain swelling and brain injury. The reason for her narrative was Death, though "It was unknown if an autopsy was performed."

But then Pfizer's investigator concludes, "there was no reasonable possibility that the cardiac arrest was related to the study intervention or clinical trial procedures, as the death occurred 2 months after receiving Dose 2. Pfizer concurred with the investigator's causality assessment."

And there are hundreds more facile dismissals of vaccine causality throughout. The wording, "no reasonable possibility that the [fill-in-the-blank symptom] was related to the study intervention," followed by "Pfizer concurred with the investigator's causality assessment," occurs 231 times in this document. There are only six instances of "Pfizer did not concur," and each of these is to overrule an investigator who suggested possible causality with Pfizer's shot or with some other medication given during the trial.

This formula was repeated with the next post-BNT162b2 death listed, that of a 60-year-old white male who died of arteriosclerosis—meaning hardening of the arteries—three days after receiving Dose 1 (p.19). "The study site received a police report indicating that the police visited the subject's home to perform a welfare check on 13 Sep 2020 (Day 4) and found him dead. It was reported that the subject's body was cold and had visible lividity. According to the medical examiner, the probable cause of death was progression of atherosclerotic disease. Relevant tests were unknown. Autopsy results were not available at the time of this report."

So again, no autopsy, even though Pfizer's *Dose-Finding Study* stipulates several times, "In the case of a participant death, a summary of available autopsy findings must be submitted as soon as possible to Pfizer Safety" (e.g., p.110).

Whitewashing Injuries

The *Narratives* document goes on to list four cases reporting a 'Serious Adverse Event' after Pfizer's BNT162b2 was injected. They are: a 30-year-old Asian female who experienced shoulder pain and decreased manual dexterity (p.26); a 53-year-old white female who suffered extreme shooting pains in her lower back and legs (p.29); a 71-year-old white female who experienced ventricular arrhythmia the day she received a second dose (p.34); and a 48-year-old white female who was diagnosed with lymphadenopathy—meaning enlarged lymph nodes—12 days after receiving Dose 1 (p.38).

In each case, the investigator thought there was a "reasonable possibility" that the symptoms were related to the "study intervention," but Pfizer agreed only with the first of these, that of the 30-year-old Asian female. In the case of the 71-year-old white female, whose heart rate surged the same day she got the second dose, and approached 200 beats per minute the following day, "Pfizer commented that there was not enough evidence to establish a causal relationship with the study intervention apart from a chronological association at this time of the report."

So thus goes Pfizer's logic. Lack of chronological association was grounds to dismiss causality for the 56-

year-old female who died of a heart attack, but the presence of chronological association was deemed irrelevant for the 71-year-old's arrhythmia.

The *Narratives* document then details 68 instances of 'Safety-Related Subject Withdrawal', the reasons ranging from heart conditions to brain injuries and cancer. One involved a 49-year-old Asian male with no pertinent medical history who had a heart attack seven days after one dose of BNT162b2 (p.124). Still, the investigator opined, "there was no reasonable possibility that the acute myocardial infarction was related to the study intervention." Naturally, "Pfizer concurred with the investigator's causality assessment."

Another Asian male, 64 years old, who also came into the study with no pertinent medical history, was diagnosed with Parkinsonism 14 days after Dose 1 (p.184). Again, the investigator deemed it unrelated to the study intervention.

There is also a death in this group, that of a 72-year-old white male (p.194), miscategorized as 'Safety-Related Subject Withdrawal'. He fainted 19 days after Dose 1 and died 16 days after that. "No reasonable possibility," said the investigator. Pfizer concurred.

The next category is 'Other Serious Adverse Event', which contains 210 cases. They include a 66-year-old white female with no pertinent medical history who was diagnosed with a stroke ('cerebrovascular accident') 32 days after Dose 2 (p.372). Again, nothing to see here, according to the investigator, and Pfizer concurred.

And the pattern of sanitization continued throughout.

The investigator would infer a link with the study intervention when it came to milder symptoms but ruled it out for severe ones.

This may have been less taxing to the investigator's conscience when the subject had an underlying condition prior to vaccination, but it seemed never to occur to them that Pfizer's medicine could reawaken or aggravate old symptoms. Even so, the post-vaccination symptoms deemed unrelated sometimes had nothing to do with the pre-existing condition. For example, an investigator declared "no reasonable possibility..." for a 77-year-old white female diagnosed with leukemia 57 days after a second dose of Pfizer (p.376). Her prior conditions, however, were drug hypersensitivity, nicotine dependence, hypertension, and osteoporosis.

Pernicious Placebos

Even more bizarrely, perhaps, the document lists four participants who died after receiving a placebo. They were: a 58-year-old white male who suffered a heart attack and died in his sleep 15 days after receiving one dose (p.10); a 51-year-old white female who died of unknown causes about a month after receiving a second dose (p.13); a 42-year-old white female who died a week after receiving a first dose, also of unknown causes (p.16); and a 61-year-old white female who was diagnosed with hemorrhagic stroke 14 days after Dose 2 and died the next day (p.22). The latter occurred in Pfizer's Argentina trials.

Among the serious adverse-event cases following placebo, a 69-year-old white female with no pertinent medical history was diagnosed with cerebral infarction 21 days after Dose 1 (p.262). This occurred in Pfizer's South Africa trials.

Another involved a 43-year-old white male with no pertinent medical history who was diagnosed with leukemia seven days after Dose 2 (p.305). The condition "was ongoing at the time of last available report and considered to be life threatening by the investigator." The investigator's concluded, however, "there was no reasonable possibility that the chronic myeloid leukemia was related to the study intervention or clinical trial procedures, but rather it was related to a genetic change in stem cells. Pfizer concurred with the investigator's causality assessment."

So, quite apart from the devastation inflicted by Pfizer's medicine, what are we to infer about the so-called 'placebos'? Were they really inert fluids that the body could, without harm, process and excrete? Were they, as defined on the CDC website, "A substance or treatment that has no effect on living beings"? Or were they a variation on the deadly BNT162b2 theme? According to researcher and former pharmaceutical executive, Sasha Latypova, in a May 2023 interview with Dr. Jane Ruby, "Placebo doesn't mean saline. In vaccine studies, they use other vaccines for placebo."

In Closing…

Pfizer's *Narratives* document bears witness to a litany of incalculable suffering caused by Pfizer's jabs in 2020 alone. Yet the deities of Big Pharma were still not satisfied, and continued to demand more human sacrifice in 2021 and beyond. How much additional suffering could have been avoided if the FDA had acted honorably and alerted the wider public to possible harms before rolling out Pfizer's deadly serum to an unsuspecting population? So much for the Hippocratic Oath!

9

TURNING US AGAINST OURSELVES: HOW PFIZER ENGINEERED AUTOIMMUNITY

Consider the position of the Allies in the Second World War. They didn't just confront the enemy in the field, and the enemy's armaments; they also attacked the munitions factories that supplied them. Any competent general would do so.

Is our immune system any less competent? Pfizer seems to think so. Its 'vaccine' technology, we are told, causes cells in the human body to produce spike proteins. Then, the theory goes, the immune system is primed to go after those spike proteins and any more it comes across. But does the immune system stop there? Or does it go after the cells that produced the spike?

'Autoimmunity' is the term used to describe such a dangerous outcome when the body attacks itself. In the words of former Pfizer executive and now whistleblower, Dr. Michael Yeadon, "Causing the body to express NON-SELF PROTEINS will automatically cause autoimmune attack on your own tissues. Why? Because your immune system is trained from before birth to recognise as foreign anything that is NOT self."

He echoes famed microbiologist, Sucharit Bhakdi, who said during a presentation in Vienna last year, "All mRNA vaccines are dangerous and are going to threaten life. It does not matter whether the vaccine encodes for the spike protein, for the measles protein, for rubella, for the flu; it does not matter at all. Why? Because the whole danger of the vaccine stems from the ability of the immune system to recognize non-self."

In Pfizer's Biological Product File, prised from the FDA through fierce legal action, the word 'autoimmune' occurs 42 times in Appendix I of Pfizer's *Cumulative Analysis* report. In a single run-on sentence spanning nine densely-typed pages, the appendix lists 1,294 'Adverse Events of Special Interest' (AESI). An AESI, according to World Health Organization guidance, "is a pre-specified medically-significant event that has the potential to be causally associated with a vaccine product."

Among the conditions preceded by the term 'autoimmune' in Pfizer's AESI list are: anaemia, arthritis, blistering, demyelination, dermatitis, diabetes, encephalopathy, endocrine disorder, eye disorder, hepatitis, hypothyroidism, inner-ear disease, lung disease, myocarditis, neuropathy, neuropsychiatric disorders, pancreatitis, pericarditis, thrombocytopenia, and thyroid disorder.

The appendix also lists two autoimmune conditions affecting male fertility, 'Anti-sperm antibody positive', where a man's immune system kills his own sperm, and 'Testicular autoimmunity'. The former is one of 49 further conditions ending with 'antibody positive', meaning again that autoimmunity is in play.

And there are catch-all terms in the list, such as 'autoimmune disorder' and 'autoimmune syndrome', along with autoimmune conditions that don't contain these terms, such as Guillain-Barre syndrome. Thus, even in Pfizer's own documents, autoimmunity is acknowledged as a major potential concern, and it appears that no part or system of the body is spared.

But what about real-world experience after Pfizer's COVID shot went into arms? Did autoimmune conditions play out then? Yes, even in the same document they did. Table 7 (p.20) of *Cumulative Analysis* tallies 1,050 cases of 'Immune-mediated/autoimmune disorders', with 12 known deaths in this category.

And these numbers are from unsolicited adverse-event reports Pfizer received between its initial emergency-use authorizations in December 2020 and the close of February 2021. This meant, in Pfizer's own words, that "the magnitude of underreporting is unknown" (p.5).

Along with Yeadon and Bhakdi, Canadian doctor, Mark Trozzi MD, is among a growing chorus of doctors sounding the alarm about autoimmune conditions. In an April 2023 interview with Odessa Orlewicz, he warned injected colleagues of "spike protein poisoning, autoimmune response, and then rabid immune dysfunction."

His message is amplified by immunologist and

virologist, Thomas Binder. "This modified RNA genocide is the greatest medical crime in human history," he said in an April 2023 video. "Its two fundamental flaws are: the injection of the construction plan for a protein foreign to the body without having any control over which body cells will produce it, in what dose, and for how long; and the fact that the cells who are coerced to produce this foreign protein, and then present it on the surface, will be mistakenly recognized by our immune system as foreign, thus destroyed, much like the rejection of a foreign organ transplanted into you. The alleged modified-RNA vaccination coerces your body to produce a toxin in unknown dose and for an unknown period of time and literally transforms parts of you into an alien. Therefore, the entire modified RNA vaccine platform must be banned immediately."

Of course, Pfizer doesn't call spike protein a 'poison'. "Turning your body into medicine factories" is the description it prefers but, as famed researcher and activist Karen Kingston points out, the 'medicine' Pfizer is referring to "is that highly inflammatory pathogen called a spike protein that causes disease, disabilities and death."

In the past few years, we have seen the COVID agenda tear society apart, even destroying marriages and families, but Pfizer would have us each of us turn even against ourselves.

10

PFIZER'S ASSAULT ON THE GENETIC CODE

"You created my inmost being," declares the Psalmist of Scripture. "You knit me together in my mother's womb." With these words, a mortal man sings his awestruck wonder at the miracle of creation, even the creation of himself.

Who, then, would dare tamper with this divine mystery? Well, Pfizer for one. In a November 2021 interview with The Atlantic Council, Pfizer's CEO Albert Bourla praised his company's 'vaccine' as a form of "gene-editing." Its technology, he asserted, could even correct mistakes in DNA.

But Pfizer didn't deem genetic alteration a worthwhile avenue of investigation in clinical trials for its COVID serums falsely called 'vaccines'. In the company's *Dose-Finding Study* document, extracted from the FDA through sustained legal action, we learn that "Genetics (specified analyses) are not evaluated in this study."

Pfizer's novel medicine, we are told, embraces a break-through technology known as 'mRNA', wherein 'm' stands for 'messenger' and 'RNA' for 'ribonucleic acid'. In another document from Pfizer's file, titled *Clinical Trial Protocol,* Pfizer describes RNA as "molecular strands which contain genetic information" (p.117).

So what genetic message does Pfizer want to send with its injections? The *Protocol* document explains, "In contrast to conventional vaccines in which the viruses are cultivated and given in killed form, RNA vaccines contain the genetic information of parts of the pathogen... In the case of a vaccination with RNA, the information for producing the antigens is carried into the body and **the body produces the antigens itself**" (p.117, emphasis added).

The implications are staggering for humanity. As food scientist and broadcaster Mike Adams put it, in his May 18, 2023 broadcast, "It's a transhumanism non-human genetic material that is infused into your body that takes over the programming of your cells and their protein-synthesis functions including, in some cases, invading the nuclei of the cells and causing permanent chromosomal alterations in each cell's nucleus, and then this causes that host body to churn out proteins which are alien to humanity."

'Gene Therapy'

When, in Pfizer's own words, its vaccine sends genetic messaging, it is hard to see why Big Pharma and its media cheerleaders would object to the term 'gene therapy' to describe this, but they do. Pfizer's mRNA rival, Moderna, admits in its Securities and Exchange Commission (SEC) filing for 2018 that "mRNA is considered a gene therapy product by the FDA," but then argues it is different because gene therapies are irreversible, whereas mRNA is "designed to not irreversibly change cell DNA."

This claim is widely ridiculed in the medical-freedom community because the purveyors of mRNA have never described an off-switch for their antigen production—specifically, the production of 'spike protein'. Furthermore, medical testing shows individuals are continuing to produce spike-protein in their bodies years after their mRNA injections.

In its own SEC filing for 2020, Pfizer acknowledged, "mRNA therapies have been classified as gene therapy medicinal products… Any product candidates we develop may not be effective, may be only moderately effective, or may prove to have undesirable or unintended side effects, toxicities or other characteristics that may preclude our obtaining marketing approval or prevent or limit commercial use."

Even if mere semantics could quell fears about permanent genetic alteration, the threat resurfaces elsewhere in Pfizer's Biological Product File. In its *Cumulative Analysis* report, among the earliest papers released by the FDA in November 2021, '1P36 gene deletion' is the very first 'Adverse Event of Special Interest' (AESI) among 1,294 listed in the document's appendix. This genetic disorder, according to *MedicineNet*, is characterized by "temper tantrums, biting, behavior problems, seizures, swallowing problems..."

An AESI, according to World Health Organization guidance, "is a pre-specified medically-significant event that has the potential to be causally associated with a vaccine product." Whether 1P36 gene deletion tells of a coming zombie apocalypse, let History reveal, but it does emphasize that Pfizer is in the gene-editing business.

Another AESI listed is 'infantile genetic agranulocytosis', a genetic disorder that causes a low white-blood-cell count. Children born with this condition, *MedicineNet* reports, "suffer frequent infections from bacteria which in the past led to death in three-quarters of cases before 3 years of age."

Cancer: The Demon in Pfizer's Vial

But the dangers of gene manipulation do not stop with these two conditions, as renowned scholar Sucharit Bhakdi M.D. points out. "The integration of any foreign gene into your chromosome can cause cancer immediately, can cause all sorts of inflammation," he told CHD.TV in a May 2023 interview, "and moreover will cause this gene to be transmitted to your offspring. You will be genetically transformed forever."

Bhakdi is not alone in warning of cancer risks from the COVID shots and even 'turbo cancer'. In another CHD.TV broadcast of Nov. 11, 2022, Canadian family doctor Charles Hoffe notes, "Over the years, a small percentage of the new cancer diagnoses would, unfortunately, be stage 4 at first diagnosis, but in my practice now, it's approximately two-thirds of all cancer diagnoses since the vax rollout are stage 4." Patients whose cancers were in remission, he added, "are flaring up after their shots... The tumors are bigger than ever. They seem to grow very aggressively, spread very aggressively, and be very resistant to treatment."

During the same broadcast, another Canadian doctor, William Makis M.D., reported on the exploding death count among jabbed physicians in Canada, including "a cluster of rapid cancers and, as you've mentioned, turbo cancers that are behaving in an absolutely unprecedented manner. They grow extremely rapidly, and they are fatal in less than a year. In some cases, they are fatal in a matter of months."

Alarming as all of this is, Pfizer's cancer plot thickens with the finding of Professor Murakami, of the Tokyo University of Science, that Pfizer's vial contains simian virus 40 (SV40), a disturbing echo of the SV40 contamination, discovered in 1960, in polio vaccines.

The SV40 virus, according to a 2004 paper, "is a known oncogenic DNA virus which induces primary brain and bone cancers, malignant mesothelioma, and lymphomas in laboratory animals," and "the major types of tumors induced by SV40 in laboratory animals are the same as those human malignancies found to contain SV40 markers."

In Closing…

If we share the Psalmist's wonder that he was seen by the eyes of the Lord before he took form,[2] surely we would never tinker with this sacred crucible of creation, much less desecrate it with experimental technology. But Pfizer's reckless eagerness to do just that speaks of a callous and deadly enemy, not just to medicine, but to all Mankind.

11

FANGS AND PHARMAKEIA: ON THE NATURE OF SPIKE PROTEIN

You've probably seen images of the spiky coronavirus that showed up in 2020 to afflict the world with a novel disease called 'COVID'. Dubbed 'SARS-CoV-2', this pernicious character is coated with prongs and resembles a Second-World-War sea mine, only far more colorful. These images are computer-generated, it turns out, not photographs, but they helped produce the intended effect —stirring the population into a frenzy of fear. The spiky bits, we are told, represent 'spike protein', also known as 'spike glycoprotein' or some variation around the letter, 'S', or 'S protein'.

Spike Harms

Spike proteins are poisonous to the human body. As early as 2007, researchers determined coronavirus spike proteins "significantly induced" 'endoplasmic reticulum'

(ER) stress, a form of cell injury that can lead to cell death. ER is associated with cancer, diabetes, and neurodegenerative diseases such as Alzheimer's, Parkinson's, and Multiple Sclerosis.

More recently, a Salk Institute study of April 2021 confirmed spike protein damages human cells and fragments mitochondria, the main energy source for cells. "The spike protein alone was enough to cause disease," the researchers reported, claiming that theirs was "the first study to show that the damage occurs when cells are exposed to the spike protein on its own."

Yet, getting the human body to produce *more* spike protein was the declared intent of Pfizer's so-called 'vaccine', purportedly to prime the immune system to recognize and attack the entire virus in future. The inherent danger of this approach prompted pediatric rheumatologist, Dr. J. Patrick Whelan, to warn in a Dec. 8, 2020 public submission to the FDA's vaccines advisory committee that this technology could "cause microvascular injury (inflammation and small blood clots called microthrombi) to the brain, heart, liver and kidneys."

Regardless, the FDA gave emergency-use authorization (EUA) to Pfizer three days later on Dec. 11, 2020 and to Moderna a week after that. In that same month of December 2020, a study appeared in nature.com that cautioned in its headline, *"The S1 protein of SARS-CoV-2 crosses the blood–brain barrier in mice."* It also showed that intravenously injected spike protein was taken up by the lungs, kidneys, liver, and spleen.

Subsequent research has only underscored the dangers. Another nature.com paper, published in March 2022, showed that administration of the "brain-infiltrating" S1 protein "induced cognitive deficit and anxiety-like behavior" in mice. "These neurological symptoms were accompanied by neuronal cell death." Was this the experimental fire Pfizer wanted to play with in humans?

Designer Spike, and 'Chimera S'

The origin of the SARS-CoV-2 spike protein is another urgent question. On Mar. 20, 2015, the University of North Carolina at Chapel Hill filed a patent application titled *Methods and Compositions for Chimeric Coronavirus Spike Proteins* (publication number WO 2015/143335 A1), where 'chimeric' means, derived from more than one species.

With Ralph Baric as the lead inventor, the patent describes "a chimeric coronavirus spike protein for treating and/or preventing a disease or disorder caused by a coronavirus infection," and it reports an antibody response in mice "immunized with S-protein-based vaccines."

The purported beneficiaries were not just rodents, however. "A subject of this invention can be a mammal, and in particular embodiments is a human, which can be an infant, a child, an adult or an elderly adult." The invention could be "administered orally, intranasally, parenterally (e.g., intravenously), by intramuscular injection, by intraperitoneal injection [into a body cavity], transdermally, extracorporeally, topically or the like."

Among the possible uses of his technology, Baric describes a "multivalent vaccine" using Chimera S, which contains regions of S proteins from other viruses, including bat viruses. This would be built on a backbone of Venezuelan Equine Encephalitis Virus (VEEV).

This research was needed, according to the paper, "to rapidly respond to new emerging diseases, especially early in the epidemic when prompt public-health intervention strategies can limit mortality and epidemic spread." This was the document's first use of the word, 'epidemic'.

Spikes and Fangs

In June 2020, Academie de sciences published a study showing that the COVID-causing spike protein "contains a motif that is homologous to that of snake neurotoxins." This means that spike proteins are similar in evolutionary origin to snake venom.

The association between spike protein and snake venom is also evident in patient symptoms. *"Like Venom Coursing Through the Body"* is the title of an August 2021 article published by the University of Arizona. It reports that the enzyme sPLA2 (secreted phospholipase A2), which "has similarities to an active enzyme in rattlesnake venom," was found in blood samples of COVID patients. At high levels, this enzyme can " 'shred' the membranes of vital organs" and "may be the most important factor in predicting which patients with severe COVID-19 eventually succumb to the virus."

The article is based on a study, published in *The Journal of Clinical Investigation,* that did biochemical analysis on 127 blood samples of COVID patients. It determined that elevations in this venom-like enzyme corresponded to increased disease severity, and was especially elevated in patients who died.

Another study, published in October 2021, sought to account for the wide range of symptoms attributed to COVID—"neurological, haemorrhagic, and thrombotic"—that defy the bounds of a normal respiratory infection. It found "toxin-like peptides, almost identical to toxic components of venoms from animals," in blood and urine samples from infected patients but never in samples from uninfected individuals.

The authors listed 36 protein sequences that mapped the venoms of various snakes—including cobras, vipers, and kraits—along with a variety of venomous sea-snail species. They cited yet another paper, published earlier that month by Cheng et al, that reported two "neurotoxin-like motifs" in the S1 spike protein of the novel coronavirus "that have peptide similarities to neurotoxins from Ophiophagus (cobra) and Bungarus genera," the krait snake.

Could spike protein, then, be a cover story for animal-venom peptides? Independent investigator and broadcaster, Bryan Ardis, argues just this in a May 2023 interview with Stew Peters. COVID symptoms are not caused by a respiratory virus, he asserts, but by venoms that cause respiratory distress. "This is a central nervous-system disease, not a respiratory illness," he told Peters.

But however we label these destructive toxins, why would Pfizer want us to produce them in our own bodies? "Human beings weren't designed to manufacture venom," Ardis continues. "Why are we injecting people with the instructions to do that?"

Ardis' observations also chime with those of Dr. Lee Merritt, a former president of the Association of American Physicians and Surgeons. "The term 'virus' in Latin means 'toxin'," she told Dr. Jane Ruby in an August 2023 interview. "So they've been poisoning us, and they call it an infectious disease."

Is it far-fetched, then, to ascribe malicious intent to Pfizer's spike-protein deployment? "Toxic by design" is the phrase coined by Dr. Mike Yeadon, a former Pfizer executive. "The companies chose to encode a particular part of the virus," he told Children's Health Defense (CHD) in a February 2023 interview. "They all chose the same part, the so-called spike protein... despite the fact there is an ample literature that says that these sort of little grappling-hook bits that stick outside of the pathogens can be dangerous."

So let's revisit Pfizer's Biological Product File, prised from the FDA through legal action. According to *VACCINE RESEARCH TEST METHOD*, released April 2023, coronaviruses comprise four structural proteins: spike (S), envelope (E), membrane (M), and nucleocapsid (N). And *2.5 Clinical Overview*, released December 2021, confirms, "among these four structural proteins, S is the key target antigen for vaccine development" (p.19).

Yeadon contends this is the most dangerous choice Pfizer could have made, despite the company's claim, in its consent leaflet issued to clinical-trial participants, that "These vaccines do not contain the whole virus, or the parts of the virus that can make you ill" (p.63).

On the contrary, Pfizer's technology is "an unguided missile," Yeadon counters, that "could land anywhere. It could land in your heart, your ovaries, your testes, your brain, and if it's taken up into those cells of those organs and started doing what the design says,... various bits of your body will start turning into a virus spike-protein manufacturing site. Well, if that spike is toxic, you should expect some toxicity in any or all of those organs in which it lands."

Another prolific voice when it comes to spike-protein dangers is independent researcher, Walter M. Chesnut. In a January 2023 article, he writes, "the underlying engine of all things spike-protein-related is repeated severe cellular injury." In another piece, he warns that no organ of the body is safe, once its cells start producing spike protein: "Your body views the cells as foreign. They are invaders, they must be destroyed. This is what happens in organ transplants." Chesnut also reports on a post-vaccination autopsy that "found spike everywhere."

Spike as a Weapon?

And if we infer harmful intent in Pfizer's injection, would the term 'bioweapon' fit? Researcher, food scientist, and broadcaster, Mike Adams, has argued this forcefully in his Health Ranger Report broadcast. "You couldn't really think of a more demonic outcome than this," he said in a May 19, 2023 episode (around 7:40), "or a demonic process to turn a human body into a factory of pure evil, which is represented in the spike protein. The spike protein is the perfect weapon against human physiology. If there were a physical manifestation of Satan in a protein form, it would be the spike protein."

From a legal perspective, the bioweapon definition brings into play federal legislation, 18 USC Ch. 10. It defines a biological weapon as "any biological agent, toxin, or delivery system for other than prophylactic, protective, bona fide research, or other peaceful purposes."

In Closing...

By now, we are used to the FDA's disclosures raising more questions than they answer, but the information gap is especially wide when it comes to spike protein, a key agent of harm both in the illness dubbed 'COVID' and in the vials conjured in response. Intentional harm is the obvious inference, especially if the snake analysis holds venom. Big Pharma then becomes culpable for not just medical assault but spiritual assault too.

12

PFIZER'S SPERM-KILLING ABORTION JAB

"We have had a habit in this country," said former Pfizer executive, Dr. Mike Yeadon, "of not ever subjecting pregnant women to experimental medical therapies or even soft cheeses. So why did the College of Obstetrics and Gynaecology lie, and advise pregnant women to go and get jabbed?... This is a murderous attack on Humanity."

Yeadon's words, spoken at a Truth-Be-Told rally in London, England on May 13, 2023, express the bewilderment of millions that, far from protecting our most precious endowment of mother and child, the medical-industrial complex set about systematically destroying it.

As of November 2023, the NHS still carried on its website a Dec. 4, 2021 press release urging pregnant women "to get jabbed." It quotes Prof. Asma Khalil, a spokesperson for the Royal College of Obstetricians and

Gynaecologists, saying, "We are very concerned about the number of pregnant women who haven't been vaccinated against COVID-19."

Khalil claimed *un*vaccinated pregnant women were *more* likely, not less likely, to have a pre-term birth or stillbirth, and concluded, "Our message is clear, COVID-19 vaccination in pregnancy is safe, it is not linked to an increased risk of miscarriage or stillbirth, and it's the best way of protecting you and your baby from the virus. We are recommending all pregnant women have their COVID-19 vaccines, including their third dose booster vaccine when they are offered it."

She was echoed in the press release by then U.K. Vaccines Minister, Maggie Throup: "The COVID-19 vaccines are safe and effective for pregnant women and I urge everyone to get their vaccines as soon as they can to secure this significant protection."

By the time of that Dec. 4, 2021 press release, however, U.K. authorities had known for at least nine months that Pfizer's jab was obliterating pregnancies. We know this because the U.K. was the second-largest source of pregnancy data gathered in Pfizer's *Cumulative Analysis* document that tallied worldwide adverse events from the shot in the opening months of its debut.[1]

Pfizer recorded 270 pregnancy cases in this report,

---

1. In most categories, the U.K. was the largest contributor of adverse-events data in Pfizer's *Cumulative Analysis* document. This may reflect the U.K.'s earlier date of temporary authorisation for Pfizer's COVID injection, on Dec. 1, 2020, compared with its emergency-use authorization of Dec. 11, 2020 in the U.S.

representing 271 potential babies because one involved twins. It did not know the outcome for 238 of these pregnancies, and a further five pregnancies were "outcome pending."

That meant Pfizer knew the outcomes for only 27 pregnancies (270 minus 238 minus 5), representing 28 potential babies, including the one set of twins. This is where the tragedy hits hard, because 26 of those pregnancies experienced "spontaneous abortion," and one resulted in "premature birth with neonatal death," ending the lives of 27 potential babies. There was but one survivor, listed as "normal outcome," among the 28 potential babies (p.12).[2]

ONLY ONE OUT OF 28 BABIES SURVIVED PFIZER'S MEDICINE!

The report's appendix also contains another warning for pregnant women because, among 1,294 'adverse events of special interest' (AESI)—meaning pre-specified medically-significant events that could be caused by a vaccine product—it lists 'Anaphylactoid syndrome of

2. This calculation is derived from the following text in Pfizer's document: "Pregnancy outcomes for the 270 pregnancies were reported as spontaneous abortion (23), outcome pending (5), premature birth with neonatal death, spontaneous abortion with intrauterine death (2 each), spontaneous abortion with neonatal death, and normal outcome (1 each). No outcome was provided for 238 pregnancies (note that 2 different outcomes were reported for each twin, and both were counted)."

pregnancy,' where amniotic fluid enters the maternal blood circulation.

Even as Pfizer was digesting the overwhelming evidence of harms caused by its product, pathologist Dr. Ryan Cole warned on Mar. 4, 2021 that COVID injections could trigger an autoimmune attack on the placenta, and he told of a friend's wife who, when seven months pregnant, miscarried just after getting her shot. We now also know, because the FDA has been legally compelled to release Pfizer's Biological Product File, that Pfizer enclosed its *Cumulative Analysis* report with a May 6, 2021 letter it sent to the FDA.

And what of the jab's impact on male fertility? In its *Participant information leaflet and declaration of consent* form (p.130), dated July 2020, Pfizer told clinical-trial participants, "Men may not donate sperm until 60 days after the last vaccination."

What were men to infer from this? That they were now walking bioweapons, toxic to any sexual partner and to any offspring that resulted? Did anyone mention this 60-day stipulation to men receiving the jab after the trials were over? Or did anyone tell them, as chronicled in *2.5 Clinical Overview*, that male clinical-trial participants before them had been afflicted with 'penile neoplasm' (a malignant lesion), 'penile squamous cell carcinoma', and 'penile infection' after getting a Pfizer shot? Or that one trial participant, as observed in another untitled document, experienced "Ejaculation disorder/ brownish ejaculation" post-injection (p.3,350)?

And what about the aforementioned list of AESIs?

Was any man told that they included 'Anti-sperm antibody positive', meaning his immune system might kill his own sperm? Or 'Penile vein thrombosis', meaning a blood clot in his penis? Or 'Testicular autoimmunity'?

We also learn from Pfizer's *Tissue Distribution Study,* conducted on rats and signed Nov. 5, 2020, that the dangerous jab components called 'lipid nanoparticles' (LNP) rapidly accumulate in the testes post-injection. The concentration increased 10-fold between 15 minutes after the jab and 48 hours (p.24), at which point the data gathering was stopped.

This study preceded by more than a month the FDA's own authorization to Pfizer in the U.S., granted on Dec. 11, 2020. Yet the medical-science community knew two years earlier that nanoparticles (NP) damage male reproductivity. A 2018 study titled *Potential adverse effects of nanoparticles on the reproductive system* noted, "NPs can cross biological barriers, including the barriers that protect reproductive tissue. Several studies have demonstrated that various NPs can pass through the blood–testis barrier (BTB) and exert their toxic actions on spermatogenesis."

The article also warns that NP accumulation "damages organs (testis, epididymis, ovary, and uterus) by destroying Sertoli cells, Leydig cells, and germ cells, causing reproductive organ dysfunction that adversely affects sperm quality, quantity, morphology, and motility or reduces the number of mature oocytes." Sertoli cells contribute to the production of sperm, Leydig cells produce testosterone and are involved in male body development, and germ cells are precursors of sperm cells.

Thus, as author Naomi Wolf observed in a Sept. 18, 2022 article, "beyond just suppressing sperm count and sperm motility, the injections damage baby boys' and small boys' and teenage boys' ability to grow up normally in terms of the development of masculinity itself."

The COVID shots have even thwarted sexual arousal and desire, according to Wolf. In a Sept. 27, 2022 interview with The Glazov Gang, she said a "metaphysical evil" was at work, that we were in "a Biblical moment" and witnessing a depopulation agenda to "poison intimacy, poison desire, poison the joy that men and women have together, make it impossible to conceive, make people barren, make it impossible for a mother to breastfeed her child, which is the most sacred and beautiful thing that is part of being female, bring babies into the world with no nurture from the mother's body."

Yet, even as Pfizer assaulted human fertility, officials clung to their denials, not just in the U.K. but glaringly so in the U.S. For example, the National Institutes of Health (NIH) issued a news release on Jan. 20, 2022 titled *COVID-19 vaccination does not reduce chances of conception, study suggests*. And the FDA's Dr. Peter Marks, ever the relentless cheerleader for Big Pharma, stated in a May 19, 2022 video, "Pregnant or breastfeeding women can certainly receive a COVID-19 vaccine... There is currently no evidence that any vaccines, including COVID-19 vaccines, cause fertility problems in either women or men."

Let us recall, then, Orwell's warning shortly before his death. "In our world," he said, "there will be no emotions except fear, rage, triumph, and self-abasement. The sex instinct will be eradicated. We shall abolish the orgasm. There will be no loyalty except loyalty to the party. But always, there will be the intoxication of power."

It is a terrifying outcome, yet one that Big Pharma has brutally served. Through its harms to reproductive capacity alone, Pfizer has sewn death for generations to come.

13

BOTCHED INJECTIONS MAGNIFY PFIZER HARMS

Our instinctive response to sharp metal objects is to keep our distance from them. Our skin being the first line of defense against external assault, we instinctively guard against its penetration, nor would we recklessly pierce the skin of another. According to one version of the Hippocratic Oath, doctors pledge not to “put a knife to” another’s flesh “if I don’t know how.”

This at least was our shared understanding until the COVID era. Time was when our bodies were regarded as sacred temples, made in the image of God, and to be respected as such but now, governments, health ministers, employers, and even travel companies consider our bodies and medical status to be their property, to be used and abused, probed and poked, exploited and exhausted at their decree, and then finally discarded as medical waste.

For statistical evidence of this, look no further than Pfizer's Biological Product File, wrested from the FDA through sustained legal action. There, quite apart from the inherent dangers of Pfizer's vile vials, we see a horrific litany of abuse in the very act of putting the poison in people's arms in the first place.

Among the earliest documents released was Pfizer's *Cumulative Analysis* report which tallies adverse events voluntarily submitted to Pfizer by Feb. 28, 2021. It records 2,792 occurrences of medication error experienced by 2,056 COVID-jab recipients (meaning some experienced more than one event). Of these, seven died, though Pfizer adds in a footnote, "the relationship between the medication error and the death is weak" (p.26, fn.3). These numbers were gleaned from voluntary reports so that, as the document states, "the magnitude of underreporting is unknown" (p.5).

But the medication errors continued piling on in the following months and years, as documented in Pfizer's third *Periodic Safety Update Report* (*PSUR #3*) to the European Medicines Agency. In Section 9.2 (starting p.102), the report tallies 68,025 cases of medication error worldwide just in its six-month reporting period of Dec. 19, 2021 to June 18, 2022. Again, these numbers rely on unsolicited reports and are therefore understated.

The first footnote on the section's opening page lists a broad range of mistakes made in administering the shots, including product administration, dispensing, distribution, dosage, expiration, exposure, labeling, preparation, prescription, selection, storage, substitution, temperature, and usage, along with "accidental poisoning." Also listed are wrong device, wrong patient, wrong product, wrong strength, and wrong technique.

Among the most frequently reported events were: "Poor quality product administered (17837 events), Product administered to patient of inappropriate age (7952 events), Product administration error (6946 events)," and "Incorrect route of product administration (1889 events)" (p.104). There were also seven cases where the subject "intentionally refused to be vaccinated or was not able to receive the scheduled BNT162b2" (p.103), and an unspecified number of "subject non-compliance" events (p.111).

Pfizer's *PSUR #3* report acknowledged harm associated with 1,398 medication-error events happening to 1,326 individuals. Two fatalities were recorded. One was an 84-year-old male who "received an incorrect fourth dose of BNT162b2 (dose unspecified) and experienced a fatal event of intestinal haemorrhage." The other was an 89-year-old female who received a second booster dose by mistake "and died due to cardiac failure and acute pulmonary oedema 2 days after the time of vaccination" (p.105).

"Serious" medication-error harms were acknowledged for 70 individuals (with 78 events), 43 of whom were in the U.K. They include 18 instances of vaccination at the wrong anatomical site and 10 incorrect routes of administration (p.106). Also tallied there are eight events of error in administration technique, including injury to nerve/blood vessel, moving the needle around in the arm, and injection with force.

Errors on Children

Dilution errors were also rampant during the *PSUR #3* reporting period, with 412 instances of "dilution before use not performed," among 1,095 instances of "incorrectly prepared vaccine." One victim seriously harmed after failure to dilute was a female child of unspecified age. "The treating nurse administered the wrong dose of vaccine to the child," the report stated. "She was supposed to dilute it, instead she gave a full vial of the COVID Vaccine (PTs: Product preparation error; Overdose). Following administration, the subject experienced dizziness, nausea, and increased heart rate. These events were considered serious as the subject requiring [sic] hospitalization and it was unknown if the subject recovered from these events. No further information was available."

PSUR #3 also tallies 51 events where children were given adult doses (p.114). A few months after the reporting period, there was another incident in Southampton, England where, in October 2022, 36 children aged five to 11 were "given a higher-than-normal dose of the Covid vaccine by mistake."

Pre-Authorization Jabs

Yet another category of error against children was injecting them before the regulatory authorities had extended authorizations down to their age group. Again, the U.K. was especially egregious in this regard, accounting for 29 of the 34 children under 12 who received premature inoculation by Feb. 28, 2021, according to Pfizer's *Cumulative Analysis* report (p.13). The ages in this group ranged from 2 months to 9 years, with a median age of four. Of the 34 cases, 24 were categorized as "serious," and 18 case outcomes were not resolved or unknown.

Yet underage injection was still frequent more than a year later. Pfizer's medicine was not authorized for six-month-olds in the U.S. until June 18, 2022, one day before the close of *PSUR #3*'s reporting period. Until then, the minimum age was five years old, but *PSUR #3* records 33 times when it was administered "to paediatric individual below 5 years of age" (p.112). The age range of those affected by medication error ranged from one month (p.105).

Fumbling Pharmacies

True to form, Pfizer concludes, at the close of its section on medication errors in *PSUR #3*, "The number and seriousness of the reported medication errors events do not indicate any trend and potential needs for any additional mitigation activity" (p.115). To the common-sense observer, however, they amount to a litany of bungling, incompetence, and indifference, the predictable result of rolling out a novel medical technology with 'Warp-Speed' abandon while cloaking the entire supply chain in legal immunity.

The prevalence of medication error also reflects the central role of pharmacies in dosing the public with Pfizer's serum. As of July 21, 2023, according to CDC, more than 305 million doses of COVID-19 vaccine had been administered in the U.S. under its Federal Retail Pharmacy Program for COVID-19 Vaccination (FRPP). "Designed to use the strength and expertise of pharmacy partners to help rapidly and conveniently vaccinate the American public," the program has 21 national pharmacy partners, including CVS, Kroger, Publix, Rite Aid, Walgreens, and Walmart, with 41,000 locations.

Also, as legal researcher Katherine Watt points out in a July 1, 2023 article, other dispensers of COVID jabs "include corporate health care 'providers' offices, paid off with escalating bounties for hitting percentage benchmarks in their patient populations, and pop-up tent or drive-through clinics located in parking lots, at businesses and at schools."

Meanwhile, the U.S. Health and Human Services Department (HHS) has provided executive cover for all this by extending Public Readiness and Emergency Preparedness (PREP) Act legal-immunity protections to an ever expanding legion of skin-piercers. On Oct. 22, 2020, several weeks before Pfizer's COVID jab was even rolled out to the public, HHS issued guidance that authorized pharmacy interns to administer childhood vaccines to patients aged three through 18 years, COVID-19 tests, and COVID-19 vaccines when made available. Furthermore, HHS decreed, "This authorization preempts any state and local law that prohibits or effectively prohibits those who satisfy these requirements from administering COVID-19 or routine childhood vaccines." In short, HHS was playing king over states' autonomy.

By the time of HHS' Eleventh Amendment to its PREP-Act Declaration for 'countermeasures' against COVID, issued May 12, 2023, liability protections for COVID injections now embraced midwives, paramedics, emergency medical technicians, physician assistants, dentists, podiatrists, optometrists, and veterinarians. Individuals in these groups would still be covered for up to five years after their licenses had lapsed.

"They wanted to make it as easy as possible," Watt observed in an August 2023 interview with Dr. Jane Ruby, "to make totally unqualified, unsupervised, untrained people able to do this work, and they do. They don't have any of the training that an actual doctor or nurse would have, to look for adverse effects or ask the person about other pre-existing conditions or other medications or anything. They have been told, 'You don't have to care about any of that. Get it in the arm, get them out within 15 minutes, and whatever happens after that, you don't need to know about, you don't need to worry about.' "

In Closing...

From start to finish, the pharmaceutical-hospital-emergency-industrial complex, to use the phrase coined by James Roguski, has carved a trail of butchery through the flesh of Man. It has swept aside all inconvenient friction to its twin agendas of profit and genocide, so that those who laid down on Big Pharma's Satanic altar also had to endure its clumsy knives.

14

PFIZER'S CHILD SACRIFICE

They sacrificed their sons and their daughters unto devils, and shed innocent blood, even the blood of their sons and of their daughters, whom they offered unto the idols of Canaan, and the land was defiled with blood.

— *PSALM* 106:37-38

When, in December 2020, Pfizer's COVID 'vaccine' gained emergency-use authorization (EUA) for adults, the company had apparently won its 'Warp-Speed' sprint to develop a countermeasure against the dreaded SARS-CoV-2 virus.

But as it turned out, this was just the first leg in a race to inject younger and younger age groups. Just five months later, on May 10, 2021, the FDA extended Pfizer's EUA down to 12-year-olds, then to five-year-olds on Oct. 29, 2021, and finally to six-month olds on June 17, 2022.

Even that did not satisfy Pfizer, as we now know from its document titled *License Action Recommendation Documents for Submissions and FDA Communication*. It shows that, in July 2021, Pfizer was in talks with the FDA about "another study to enroll infants <6 months of age" (p.10).

Indirect Harms to Children

Pfizer didn't entirely get its way, though, because the EUAs stopped at six-month-olds, but it managed to target even younger victims anyway, either in the womb or at the breast of their injected mothers. We know this from Pfizer's *Cumulative Analysis* document that tallied worldwide adverse-event reports in the opening months of vaccine authorizations. Like the aforementioned *License Action* document, it is part of Pfizer's Biological Product File extracted from the FDA through sustained legal action.

... in the womb.

Based on reports Pfizer received from 63 countries between December 2020 and the close of February 2021, the *Cumulative Analysis* document tallied 270 pregnancy cases, representing 271 potential babies because one involved twins. Pfizer did not know the outcome for 238 pregnancies, and a further five pregnancies were "outcome pending."

That meant Pfizer knew the outcomes for only 27 pregnancies (270 minus 238 minus 5), representing 28 potential babies, including the one set of twins. This is where the tragedy hits hard, because 26 of those 27 pregnancies experienced "spontaneous abortion," and there was one instance of "premature birth with neonatal death."

THUS, 27 OF THE 28 POTENTIAL BABIES DIED. THERE WAS BUT ONE SURVIVOR, LISTED AS "NORMAL OUTCOME."

These numbers, devastating as they are, represent but a sample of the total because, as the document notes, "Reports are submitted voluntarily, and the magnitude of underreporting is unknown" (p.5).

The same applies to Pfizer's *Periodic Safety Update Report (PSUR #1)*, spanning 286 pages, to the European Medicines Agency (EMA). Covering the six-month period from Dec. 19, 2020 through June 18, 2021, this 'pharmacovigilance' document is supposed to detect safety signals based on adverse-event data both from Pfizer's clinical trials and from its post-authorization rollouts. These are listed separately. The report was not publicly released until early 2023 after an unnamed researcher obtained it via FOIA request and provided it to TKP, an Austrian blog.

PSUR #1 records 1,604 pregnant-mother cases in its

post-authorization data, of which 945 led to adverse events. The serious events with nine occurrences or more were: "Abortion spontaneous (275), Vaginal haemorrhage (27), Abortion missed (21), Foetal death (16), Abortion (9)" (p.241). In addition, there were seven elective pregnancy terminations, of which six were due to "foetal defects" (p.242).

Pfizer's *third Periodic Safety Update Report (PSUR #3)* to the EMA, covering the year-later period (Dec. 19, 2021 to June 18, 2022) added a further 566 spontaneous-abortions from 1,898 known pregnancy outcomes, and 78 cases of vaginal haemorrhage (p.336). There were 23 elective pregnancy terminations, 22 of which were "due to foetal defects," with the reason for the one remaining termination unknown (p.337).

Among the infants born alive, 31 infants were born with congenital anomalies, including cardiac disorder, chromosome abnormality, growth restriction, kidney malformation, congenital amputation, and congenital disorders of foot, hand, limbs, and spine.

... at the breast.

Even then, babies were not safe from indirect vaccine injury, as those who survived 'transplacental' harms were then in danger of 'transmammary' harms through breast milk that contained vaccine products from injected mothers. There were early warning signs of this in Pfizer's *Cumulative Analysis* document, which noted one case of suppressed lactation and one of breast-milk discoloration.

Shortly after, reports of infant deaths from tainted breast milk started appearing in the Vaccine Adverse Events Reporting System (VAERS), a database jointly managed by the FDA and the CDC. The earliest reports include...

- A breast-feeding five-month-old boy who died soon after his mother got a second Pfizer dose on March 17, 2021. The next day, he "developed a rash and within 24 hours was inconsolable, refusing to eat, and developed a fever. Patient brought baby to local ER where assessments were performed, blood analysis revealed elevated liver enzymes. Infant was hospitalized but continued to decline and passed away. Diagnosis of TTP. No known allergies. No new exposures aside from the mother's vaccination the previous day" (VAERS ID: 1166062).

- A one-year-old boy who went into intense febrile seizures on Feb. 19, 2021 after "vaccine exposure via breast milk." His mother had received a first Pfizer dose four days earlier (VAERS ID: 1161763).

- A six-week-old boy who died on July 17, 2021 "from clots in his severely inflamed arteries," as

> reported to VAERS by his 36-year-old mother. "I had been breastfeeding my 6 week old baby at the time that I received the first Pfizer vaccine... I am curious if the spike protein could have gone through the breast milk and caused an inflammatory response in my child" (VAERS ID: 1532154).

Many more such cases are cited in a *NewsRescue* article of Sept. 22, 2021. It also notes, "A number of reports describe mothers' milk drying up suddenly after vaccination."

Transmammary harms snowballed further in Pfizer's PSURs to the EMA. The cases are harder to tease out from these large documents, but they include 61 cases deemed 'serious' in *PSUR #1* (p.245) and a further 66 serious cases in *PSUR #3* (p.340). Elsewhere, the documents list two cases of stroke among breastfeeding infants (*PSUR #1*, p.163), three neurological cases (*PSUR #1*, p.149), and four respiratory cases (*PSUR #3*, p.239).

That vaccine contents make their way to breast milk was also demonstrated in a study published September 2022 in *JAMA Pediatrics*. It found that, among 11 lactating women, trace amounts of Pfizer and Moderna vaccine contents were detected in the breast milk of five women within 45 hours of receiving a vaccination (Table 2).

So what did Pfizer conclude after such a litany of harm in the PSURs? That "There were no safety signals regarding use in pregnant/lactating women that emerged from the review of these cases or the medical literature" (*PSUR #3*, p.340). Naturally, the various regulatory authorities rubber-stamped Pfizer's self-serving analysis, and the public were none the wiser.

How did Pfizer achieve this sleight of hand? Sometimes, it would cite prior medical conditions in the mother, or her lifestyle choices, as contributing factors in harms to mother or child; occasionally, it cited the mother's advanced age for childbearing; but most of the time, Pfizer resorted to "limited information regarding the mother's obstetric history, which precluded meaningful causality assessment" (e.g., *PSUR #3*, p.331).

... from injected parents.

Yet another vector of danger for young children is to receive secondhand vaccine contents from jabbed parents, whether via inhalation or skin contact. Since 2001, microscopy analysis has shown disturbing structures in blood samples taken from the injected, but then similar structures started appearing in the uninjected who had been in close proximity to jab recipients. These effects have proven especially harmful in children.

Dr. Philippe van Welbergen, a U.K.-based physician, has been foremost in sounding the alarm. In a February 2022 presentation, he showed a blood sample from an unjabbed eight-year-old child who became partially paralyzed after their blood was devastated by transmitted injection components (around 1:14:30).

Direct Harms to Children

And what of children given the needle itself? The *Cumulative Analysis* report alone gave early and ample warning of what lay ahead. No child was supposed to receive a Pfizer shot during the reporting period, which ended Feb. 28, 2021, but Pfizer knew of 34 children aged between two months and nine years who did. Twenty-nine of them were in the U.K. Of the 34 children, 24 experienced at least one serious adverse event (p.13).

Table 7 of the report also details two childhood-injury cases reported to Pfizer by the U.K. Medicines and Healthcare products Regulatory Agency (MHRA, p.25). The first "described a 1-year-old subject who received the vaccine, and had left postauricular ear pain that progressed to left-sided Bell's palsy 1 day following vaccination that had not resolved at the time of the report." Another "described a 7-year-old female subject who received the vaccine and had stroke (unknown outcome); no follow-up is possible for clarification."

Yet Pfizer's paper concludes, "No new significant safety information was identified based on a review of these cases compared with the non-paediatric population" (p.13). Should we be comforted by this language, telling us the outcomes for children were no worse than the outcomes for adults? Not when the document counted 1,223 post-injection deaths among all age groups (p.7) among 42,086 individuals who experienced between them 158,893 events.

Then the document's appendix (p.30) lists 1,294

adverse events of special interest (AESI), meaning pre-specified medically-significant events that could be caused by the vaccine product. These include 'Child-Pugh-Turcotte score abnormal' (signalling liver disease), 'Convulsion in Childhood', 'Multisystem inflammatory syndrome in children', and 'Paediatric autoimmune neuropsychiatric disorders associated with streptococcal infection'.

Again, Pfizer's PSURs to the EMA darken the horrors still further, with *PSUR #3* logging 161 post-authorization fatalities among under-18s in the cumulative data set (combining all PSURs to date) (p.292). These deaths were tied to 339 adverse events (meaning there could be multiple adverse events for one individual), with 78 categorized as cardiac disorders, 56 as nervous-system disorders, and 62 as respiratory, thoracic, and mediastinal (p.293).

The top 5 MedDRA SOCs with the most frequently reported (>3000 occurrences) events with a fatal outcome cumulative by age group in the PM data are presented in the table below.

Table 66. Post-Authorisation Data: Total Number of AEs with a Fatal Outcome by SOCs and by Age Group - Cumulative Reporting Interval

SOC	Total number of events	≤ 17 years	18-24 years	25-49 years	50-59 years	60-69 years	70+ years	Unk
General disorders and administration site conditions	8735	115	65	612	534	956	5720	733
Cardiac disorders	5014	78	59	539	433	700	3075	130
Nervous system disorders	3818	56	63	336	311	516	2433	103
Respiratory, thoracic and mediastinal disorders	3535	62	32	282	251	444	2395	69
Infections and infestations	3473	28	21	108	118	355	2596	247

Of note, multiple AEs may be reported in a single case.

Five- through 11-year-olds.

PSUR #3 then segments the pediatric data by age group. It records 20 post-authorization deaths among 9,605 injured individuals aged five through 11 years old in its six-month reporting period (p.321).

One death involved an 11-year-old boy who went into acute respiratory failure two days after his first dose of Pfizer's 'BNT162b2' vaccine. No autopsy was performed. Another was a six-year-old girl whose fatal adverse events included kidney impairment and seizure. She died seven days after her first dose. It was unknown whether an autopsy was performed. A six-year-old boy died with myocarditis and cardio-respiratory arrest seven days after his first dose, though "the reporter concluded that the death 'had nothing to do' with the administration of BNT162b2 and was due to natural causes." Autopsy results were pending.

Among the remaining fatal cases, cardiac and respiratory events were the main killers. Cerebral haemorrhage, multisystem inflammatory syndrome, and pulmonary embolism were also among the reported events (p.322).

12- through 17-year-olds.

Among 12- through 17-year-olds, *PSUR #3* tallies 62 fatal cases post authorization in its six-month reporting interval. Here, Pfizer made a very rare concession to possible causation, though only for 20 of the 62 deaths, for which "a causality between the vaccination and the occurrence of the fatalities cannot be ruled out, based on the temporal relationship, although no laboratory data or autopsy results provided evidence of a causal relationship."

Pfizer provided more detail on six of the deaths where it cited "underlying medical conditions" as a possible factor. A 16-year-old girl died of dyspnea three days after first dose, not known if autopsy performed. Another 16-year-old girl experienced brain injury and acute cardiac failure six days after first dose. She died suddenly of cardiac failure 35 days later, no autopsy performed. A third 16-year-old girl died of pulmonary embolism and cardiac arrest after third dose, autopsy performed but results not provided. A 13-year-old girl experienced chest pain and palpitations five days after first dose. She went into cardiac arrest and lost consciousness two months later. An autopsy was performed and determined that her death was possibly related to the vaccine.

A 17-year-old boy died of cardiac failure 92 days after second dose. The autopsy results were heavily redacted. And a 13-year-old boy died of brain death within one month of unknown dose number, not known if autopsy performed.

PSUR #3 also gives insight into the psychological toll inflicted by Pfizer's medicine, with two suicide attempts among 15 individuals harmed in the 12-17 age group during clinical trials within the six-month period (p.323).

Yet Pfizer concluded after all this, "No new significant safety information was identified based on the review of the cases reported in the overall paediatric population" (p.328).

Myocarditis.

Bear in mind that the heart events described in *PSUR #3*, many of them fatal, occurred some six months or more after the CDC's Advisory Committee on Immunization Practices (ACIP) acknowledged "reports of myocarditis and pericarditis in mRNA vaccine recipients" in a July 2021 update, but it continued to recommend "that all persons aged ≥12 years receive a COVID-19 vaccine." Its benefits, the committee maintained, "clearly outweigh the risks in all populations, including adolescents and young adults."

In June 2022, *Journal of Pediatrics* published a study from Seattle Children's Hospital reporting that over a nine-month period, 35 patients younger than 18 years of age presented with chest pain within one week of receiving a second Pfizer dose. All were diagnosed with myopericarditis, meaning inflammation of both the heart muscle and its lining.

The report presented findings on 16 of those patients who had both acute-phase and follow-up cardiac MRIs available for review. There were 15 boys in the group and one girl, and the median age was 15 years. Median time to presentation after the second Pfizer dose was three days. All patients had elevated serum troponin levels, indicating "increased risk of heart attack," and all initial cardiac MRIs were abnormal.

In follow-up MRIs, conducted between three and eight months later, 11 of the 16 patients had persistent late gadolinium enhancement (LGE), signifying ongoing myocarditis and could be "predictive of a poor outcome." LGE, the paper went on to explain, "is an indicator of cardiac injury and fibrosis... Yang et al found that presence of LGE is a predictor of all-cause death, cardiovascular death, cardiac transplant, rehospitalization, recurrent acute myocarditis, and requirement for mechanical circulatory support."

Seizures.

Another journal, *Pediatrics*, published a study in June 2023 titled *Safety of COVID-19 mRNA Vaccination Among Young Children in the Vaccine Safety Datalink*, where Vaccine Safety Datalink is a collaboration between CDC and eight data-contributing health systems in the U.S. From 135,005 Pfizer doses given to children aged six months to four years, the study reported 38 seizure events within three weeks of any dose and a further 24 seizure events in weeks four through six after most recent dose (Table 2).[1]

The authors rejoiced, however, that they "did not detect a safety signal for any outcome during the 21 days after vaccination" while omitting days 22-42 in this assessment. These results, they concluded, "can provide

---

1. From 112,006 Moderna doses, the study recorded 23 seizure events within three weeks of injection, and a further 19 seizure events in weeks four through six, for children aged six months to five years.

reassurance to clinicians, parents, and policymakers alike."

Maddie de Garay

Horrifying as all these numbers are, they do not describe the heartbreak of parents who would rue the day they brought their loved ones in to get an experimental injection. Among those parents are Stephanie and Patrick de Garay. Their daughter, Maddie, was a healthy 12-year-old girl until, on Jan. 20, 2021, she received a second Pfizer dose in clinical trials for adolescents at Cincinnati Children's Hospital.

About 18 hours after, Maddie developed severe nerve pain, a feeling like electric shocks going down her neck and spine, excruciating abdominal pain, and severe chest pain that felt like her heart was being pulled out. Her vaccine arm swelled up and became numb. Her fingers and toes turned white, and were ice cold to the touch. The pain in her toes was so bad that she had to walk on her heels.

Stephanie and Patrick took Maddie to the ER at Cincinnati Children's Hospital where they screened her for appendicitis and ruled it out. Though they found dilated loops of bowel on X-ray, and observed blood in her urine, they sent her home.

Over the following months, Maddie's condition worsened, including food regurgitation and vomiting, until she was unable to swallow any food or liquids, and had to resort to a feeding tube. The total body pain and severe abdominal pain persisted, and her abdomen became distended. She experienced fainting spells which developed into seizures, sometimes 10 a day.

Prior to injection, Maddie had never menstruated, but on Feb. 5, 2021, she started to discharge brown fluid, which came out in chunks over the following month. Painful cysts developed on her vagina and then her head. Erratic blood pressure and heart rate were also among the symptoms, along with tinnitus, vision problems, headaches, dizziness, and memory loss. Finally, she lost feeling from the waist down, which led to paralysis and incontinence.

Maddie went to the ER eight more times as her health continued to decline, until she was admitted to Inpatient Rehabilitation at Cincinnati Children's Hospital on Apr. 13, 2021. There she remained for several weeks through her 13th birthday.

A dysfunctional diagnosis.

By now, Maddie was traumatized by her experiences with doctors, who refused to believe her or acknowledge the injection triggered her symptoms. They treated her like a mental patient instead, using the facile diagnosis of 'functional neurological disorder'. After that, they stopped any further testing.

Any diagnosis that includes the word 'functional' invites skepticism. As observed by Jessica Wallace of law firm, Siri & Glimstad, an attorney with a background in vaccine-injury cases and medical malpractice, "This is a diagnosis of exclusion, and basically, they are saying it's all in the patient's head." The term also infects future diagnoses and treatments by encouraging doctors to write off patients and their symptoms with mental or behavioral labels.

One glaring example of the medical indifference Maddie endured came from Amal Hallim Assa'ad, M.D. at Cincinnati Children's. She conducted just one 15-minute consultation with Maddie on Mar. 5, 2021, but deemed this sufficient to rule out further tests. "It drives the patient to thinking that there must be something wrong that is indicating all this workup," Assa'ad wrote in her notes "It also delays the necessary psychological intervention that is needed to help resolve the functional disorder." The hospital then tried to discharge Maddie to a facility for eating disorders.

Furthermore, the misdiagnosis was formalized as 'abdominal pain' in the safety-evaluation data Pfizer turned over to the FDA as it sought authorization for its prized serum. Even that one symptom was viciously understated, as Maddie would scream in agony from that one symptom alone. On Feb. 28, 2021, from an adjoining room, Stephanie recorded her daughter crying out, "I can't do this. I can't do it. I'm gonna die. God, why are you doing this?!"

But then there was more insult added to Maddie's injury as Pfizer refused to cover her staggering medical bills. This devastating news came in a May 17, 2021 phone conversation with Dr. Robert Frenck, principal investigator for the clinical trial. The costs would not be covered, he told Patrick and Stephanie, because they were not deemed "research related"—in other words, not attributable to the trial. "The doctors that have seen her so far have not found something where they thought it was research related," he said, "is what they were all telling me."

Patrick was astonished. "Within a 24-hour period, all this went down," he said, "so if that's your stand, I find it hard to believe that you're trying to steer away from that." He tried to restrain himself as he continued, "Don't worry about my daughter can't walk or anything. As you can tell, Dr. Frenck, I'm a little upset."

Nevertheless, Frenck continued to insist the costs would be the family's responsibility, a clear and egregious breach of international law, specifically the *Declaration of Helsinki—Ethical Principles for Medical Research Involving Human Subjects*. Para. 15 states, "Appropriate compensation and treatment for subjects who are harmed as a result of participating in research must be ensured."

But Frenck was not done. Just 10 days later, he appeared as lead author on a *New England Journal of Medicine* article, published May 27, 2021, reporting on Pfizer's vaccine trial for adolescents, in which Maddie participated. Pfizer's vaccine "had a favorable safety and side-effect profile," he asserted. "There were no vaccine-related serious adverse events and few overall severe adverse events."

Pfizer's whitewash shows up in *PSUR #1*, in the section showing clinical-trial data for children aged 12 to 15. It records that 14 children experienced adverse events, with one occurrence of 'Abdominal pain'. The full list comprises "Depression (4), Suicidal ideation (3), Appendicitis (2), Abdominal pain, Anal abscess, Anxiety, Constipation, Conversion disorder, Femur fracture and Focal peritonitis (1 each). All events were assessed as unrelated to BNT162b2 or blinded therapy" (p.228).

Rogue Regulators

So how did regulators respond to all of this? The FDA had in its possession Pfizer's *Cumulative Analysis* report by May 2021 at the latest, as Pfizer's letter enclosing it is dated May 6, 2021. Its tidings of 1,223 deaths were reason enough to pull Pfizer's vile vials from every hospital, clinic, care home, and pharmacy in the world. In the words of renowned cardiologist and epidemiologist, Dr. Peter McCullough, in a Dec. 7, 2021 interview with DarkHorse Podcast, "Our vaccine program would have been shut down in January [2021] for excess mortality."

Yet the FDA's damage control was not to protect the lives of children but to protect the image of vaccines. Thus, Peter Marks, director of the FDA's Center for Biologics Evaluation and Review (CBER), told a June 29, 2021 FDA 'stakeholder call' that child deaths post-vaccination had been "very sensationalized" and were attributable to a "definitively different cause of death." He admitted that post-vaccine myocarditis was "about five times higher than the baseline" in males aged 12 to 17, but these cases had "generally been mild."

Adolescents were not going into heart failure, Marks

said, but "may have a twinge of chest discomfort." Vaccines could trigger "a somewhat exuberant immune response... that causes a little bit of inflammation in the heart. In this case, it appears to be relatively brief. Again, goes away on its own."

Mark's presentation estimated COVID vaccines led to 56-69 cases of myocarditis per million males aged 12 to 17, but he deemed this a fair price to pay for the two COVID deaths he said were prevented by injecting a million boys. He had "no hesitation whatsoever about this recommendation," even for those with pre-existing heart conditions. "Getting your child vaccinated now is something that is going to be good to do," he added, and two shots were better than one because "generally, the immunity after natural infection tends to wane after about 90 days. And we do know that the immunity after vaccination is better than the immunity after natural infection."

More perception management would be required, however, as the FDA extended Pfizer's gift (at least in the German sense of the word) to younger and younger children. On Apr. 26, 2022, Marks appeared in an FDA video—one of many in a nauseating series titled *Just a Minute!*—to promote COVID jabs for kids under five years of age. It was very troubling, he said, that only 27% of children five through 11 had been vaccinated against COVID, but he assured parents the FDA would be "thorough and transparent in our evaluations... without sacrificing our standards."

The outcome of these evaluations, however, was a

foregone conclusion. Marks continued, "Once our reviews have been completed, we will bring the vaccines before our independent advisory committee to have a transparent discussion of the data, so that when we make a determination to authorize the vaccines in young children, parents can be confident in their decision to vaccinate."

On Apr. 29, just three days later, Marks followed up with another *Just a Minute!* in which he promised the FDA would "not cut any corners" in evaluating shots for the under-fives. He didn't have to wait long because, as we have seen, the FDA extended its EUA to six-month-olds for both Pfizer and Moderna on June 17, 2022. At the following press conference, Marks asserted that the vaccines were "safe and effective for use in our nation's youngest children."

Reading from a teleprompter, he continued, "The FDA was acutely aware of the trust bestowed on it by the American people." Parents, caregivers, and health-care providers could "trust that both of these vaccines have been authorized with science and safety at the forefront of our minds." He closed by urging "individuals of all ages to get vaccinated and boosted when eligible if you've not done so already."

The following day, Rochelle Walensky, then director of the CDC, dutifully applauded in a tweet, "We now know based on rigorous scientific review that the vaccines available here in the United States can be used safely and effectively in children under 5."

Last Throw of the Dice: 'Bivalent' Boosters.

Even so, Pfizer's race had one more lap to go. Just 11 days after the FDA extended EUAs to six-month-olds, the FDA's Vaccines and Related Biological Products Advisory Committee (VRBPAC) met on June 28, 2022 to discuss 'bivalent' COVID shots, which purportedly addressed more than one virus 'variant'.

Children were in the crosshairs yet again. Dr. Mark Sawyer, for example, said he didn't want the rollout to be "too late" to address a predicted wave of new COVID infections in the Fall. Though he acknowledged "concern about side-effects and serious side-effects in children," he urged, "We are unlikely to learn about those during any clinical trials, so I think—myocarditis in particular—we're only going to know that when we roll out the vaccine, and the safety systems do their review" (around 8:09:00).

Sawyer was then echoed by Dr. Amanda Cohen who called for haste in future authorizations for children under five, saying, "I don't want concerns about myocarditis to increase the amount of time it takes to get a vaccine available for this age group" (at 8:10:10).

No surprise, then, that on Aug. 31, 2022, about a week after receiving requests from Pfizer and Moderna, the FDA authorized Pfizer's new 'updated boosters' for individuals 12 years old and up, and Moderna's for 18 and up. Both bivalent brews were later authorized to six-month-olds on Apr. 18, 2023, just in time for the official "End of COVID-19 Public Health Emergency" on May 11, 2023.

In Closing...

What motive, then, shall we attribute to Big Pharma's ruthless campaign of violence against children? According to investigative reporter, Lara Logan, the assault is as much spiritual as physical. "For them, the younger you are, the closer you are to God, the more pain they can inflict on God," she explained in a June 2022 interview with Vigilant Fox. "So the more you can make a baby or a small child suffer, the greater your victory over God. And that is the only consideration for them."

From this perspective, Pfizer is not just a corrupt corporation counting the dollars but a rapacious priesthood counting the bodies. The younger its sacrificial victims, the greater its prestige before medical deities. What else can explain its wanton slaughter of children, not just in the cradle, but in the womb and at the breast, and all at industrial scale. If, as the Bible warns, "The wages of sin are death," how much more so when the sins are against the child?

15

PFIZER'S HARVEST OF DEATH

How many deaths does it take to stop a lethal medical intervention? "Our vaccine program would have been shut down in January [2021] for excess mortality," said famed cardiologist, Dr. Peter McCullough, in a milestone interview with the DarkHorse Podcast in December 2021.

But the COVID shots would have been shut down earlier still, even before they began, if regulators had headed off the adverse events they knew were coming. On Oct. 22, 2020, seven weeks before the FDA authorized Pfizer's jab for 'emergency use' in adults, the FDA's Steven Anderson listed Death as a possible adverse event in his presentation to the FDA's Vaccines and Related Biological Products Advisory Committee (VRBPAC) (at 2:33:40 and glossed over in the blink of an eye).

Anderson's slides included a *Working list of possible adverse event outcomes* (Slide 17), which reads like a blueprint for the horrors that were to unfold. The meeting included Dr. Marion Gruber, then director of the FDA's Office of Vaccines Research & Review (appearing around 00:33:23) and Dr. Peter Marks, director of the FDA's Center for Biologics Evaluation and Research (around 1:57:00).

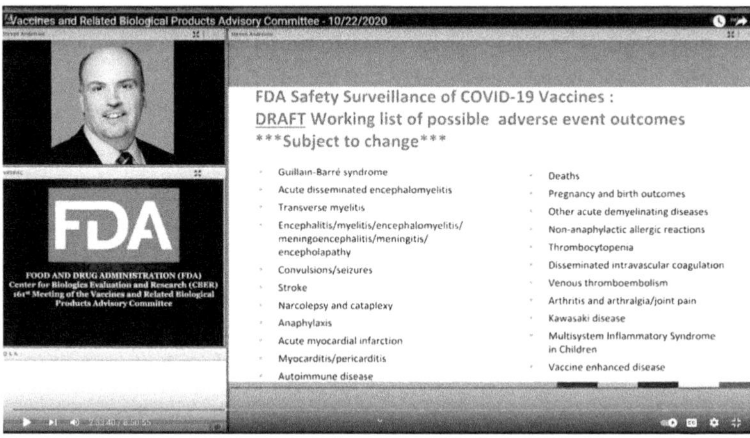

Yet here we are. Going into the winter of 2023, the COVID vaccines are still on offer, not just to adults somehow oblivious to the catastrophic harms they have inflicted worldwide, but to infants as young as six months old after a rogue FDA kept extending 'emergency-use authorization' to younger and younger cohorts.

Even official databases, such as the Vaccine Adverse Events Reporting System, cry out against the genocidal agenda perpetrated by official medicine, and that's after the numbers have been heavily suppressed and rigged by a medical bureaucracy desperate to minimize the appearance of harm.

But one number—1,223—has been quoted more than

any other in medical freedom circles. That's how many unsolicited reports of death Pfizer received within the first three months of worldwide authorizations that began in December 2020. It comes from Pfizer's *Cumulative Analysis* report to the FDA (p.7), which was in the FDA's possession by May 2021 at the latest. This grim total was gleaned from voluntary reports so that, as the document states, "the magnitude of underreporting is unknown" (p.5).

By now, we've all seen the videos of athletes dropping on the fields, pitches, and courts of sports arenas, news presenters collapsing on camera, and entertainers dropping on stage. And the phrase 'Sudden Death' daily fills the headlines. The official response, of course, is to tell us we're not seeing what we're seeing, to explain it away, and to deploy a vast censorship-industrial-complex against anyone who publicly connects the obvious dots.

But the truth-suppression efforts are wearing thin. Even official data is confirming the witness of our eyes, whether prised from regulators through legal action, supplied by whistleblowers, or dug up by Internet sleuths. Another blow to official denials has come from release of Pfizer's Periodic Safety Update Reports (PSUR) to the European Medicines Agency. The third report (*PSUR #3*) tallies 13,509 reported deaths up to June 18, 2022, and that's excluding a further 492 fatalities omitted on the grounds "death was mentioned as incidental information only" (p.291). Again, these numbers rely on passive data collection, so that the true cull is unknown.

Autopsy results were provided in 725 cases, with heart conditions accounting for the largest toll. The most commonly reported causes were: "Pulmonary embolism (82), Pulmonary oedema (61), Arteriosclerosis (54), Myocardial infarction (50), Arteriosclerosis coronary artery (48), Acute myocardial infarction (46), Myocarditis (39), Cardiac hypertrophy (33), and Cardiomegaly (31)" (p.292).[1]

Most horrifying of all, 161 paediatric deaths (17 and under) were reported up to June 18, 2022 (p.292), but Pfizer's conclusion after all this was, "No new risks were identified following review of fatal cases." Furthermore, all these deaths were on top of 76 fatalities in clinical trials alone (p.291), though Pfizer's trial investigators deemed none of the fatal events were related to the injection that preceded them.

Excess-death statistics are a further source of embarrassment for politicians and bureaucrats. Do a search on "excess deaths" at *The Exposé*, and you will find dozens of statistically rigorous articles highlighting the genocidal surge that coincided with 'vaccine' rollout. They include...

- *632x increase in Child Excess Deaths across Europe*
- *2 Million Excess Deaths across the West*
- *Ex-NZ PM Jacinda Ardern's COVID Dictatorship caused 3203% increase in Excess Deaths due to Mandatory C-19 Vaccination Laws*

- *Secret Australian Government Data confirms the Country suffered a devastating 5162% increase in Excess Deaths in 2022 compared to the height of the COVID Pandemic in 2020*

So, to answer the original question, no amount of death will put a stop to Pfizer's infernal medical interventions. Worse than mere indifference to the harm of others—the very definition of a psychopath—today's medical establishment is wielding so-called vaccines as a lethal weapon to kill and maim far and wide and, if they can get away with it, in perpetuity. So, what secret oath do the practitioners serve that they can so readily desecrate the Hippocratic Oath? And what atrocities have they committed in secret to prepare for the ones they now commit in public?

1 To the extent data was available, *PSUR #3* also lists for its six-month reporting period the number of vaccine doses administered before the subjects' deaths. First dose accounted for 378 cases, second dose for 934, third dose for 1,084, and fourth dose for 71. There was one fifth-dose case, a man who had two Coronavac jabs followed by three BNT162b2. He died three days after the final dose. "Oxygen deficiency and failure of the lungs to function were cited as the cause of death."

16

PFIZER'S MINDFUCKERY: HOW THE COVID SHOT ATTACKS HUMAN CONSCIOUSNESS

You've no doubt heard about the gas-lighting doctors inflict on injection-injured patients, attributing their life-altering and often life-ending symptoms to anything but the accursed COVID jab, but how much easier is their Pharma-shielding mission when patients report they have been psychologically harmed?

Famed microbiologist, Sucharit Bhakdi, has diligently sounded the alarm about this category of injury, telling a conference in September 2022, "All your personality is being changed. Your brain is being changed, and your heart is being weakened."

The vaccine contents, he explains, cross the blood-brain barrier, resulting in spike-protein formation and micro-clotting in brain capillaries. "Dementia, Alzheimer's, is very often associated with microclots and micronecrosis in the frontal brain... So you cannot afford to clog any single capillary in the brain. If you do this, there's going to be consequences that are irreversible."

In the subsequent Q&A, Bhakdi added, "We see our neighbors around us and say, 'My God, his mind is crumbling. He's getting stupid.' It's really true. And the will is broken; they have no will. So people are becoming enslaved animals." Bhakdi compared this to the Eloi in H.G. Wells' *The Time Machine,* a docile, incurious race who own nothing and are easy prey for the brutal, darkness-dwelling Morlocks (Day 2, Panel 7).

Bhakdi is far from alone in warning about brain damage. "The building literature on neuropsychiatric symptoms is alarming," commented Dr. Peter McCullough in a January 2023 article. He cited evidence of spike protein in the human brain after vaccination and a May 2022 paper from University Hospital in Split, Croatia that reported "acute psychotic symptoms following the administration of the COVID-19 vaccine."

The paper describes three male patients—none of whom had any past or family history of mental illness—who developed psychotic disorders following COVID-19 vaccination. Two of them, a 41-year-old and a 35-year-old, had received the Pfizer jab. The former had begun to experience frontal headaches five days after his second dose, along with paresthesias on the left side of his body, paranoid delusions, and severe anxiety.

The 35-year-old also experienced headaches and paresthesia, in this case within three days of receiving a first dose of Pfizer's BNT162b2. "He also had syncope and was examined by a neurologist, who found no deficit.

Two weeks later, he visited the psychiatric emergency room twice because of persecutory delusions and delusions of reference."

Similar vaccine effects have been documented in other medical papers. One describes a woman in her 20s who presented to an emergency department one week after receiving a first Pfizer dose. Her symptoms were acute psychosis, anxiety, decreased mental acuity, aphasia (a language disorder), auditory hallucination, and "delusions which progressed to psychosis and catatonia." During a second emergency visit, "the patient removed her clothing and had a bowel movement on the floor."

This "constellation of symptoms," the authors report, "led to a strong clinical suspicion of an autoimmune-mediated encephalitis driven by the vaccine." They urged "serious consideration of organic nervous system causes of psychosis" and concluded that psychiatric clinical presentations warrant a thorough medical workup and a vaccine history.

Another paper describes a 31-year-old male brought to an emergency room by police because of erratic and bizarre behavior. He reported "becoming 'clairvoyant', being able to talk with dead people." His symptoms began "after receiving the first dose of an mRNA-based COVID-19 vaccine, and markedly worsened three weeks later after receiving the second dose. Previously, he was asymptomatic, working full-time as an office manager." Tomography and MRI scans showed "hyperintensities throughout the subcortical and periventricular white matter."

Pfizer's Biological Product File, wrested from the jealous clutches of the FDA through legal action, lists 42 types of psychiatric disorder reported by participants during its clinical trials alone, including anxiety, depression, disorientation, insomnia, nightmare, panic attack, and sleep disorder. We also see, in Pfizer's *third Periodic Safety Update Report (PSUR #3)* to the European Medicines Agency, that there were 10 completed suicides in clinical trials alone up to June 18, 2022 (p.291).

One vector for brain damage is degradation of the myelin sheath around nerves caused by lipid nanoparticles (LNP) in the shots. The result, as described by author and activist, Naomi Wolf, is "all the things that happen when human neurological systems are degraded," including dementia, Parkinson's disease, and multiple sclerosis. The passage of LNPs through the blood-brain barrier, she surmised in an interview with international rights lawyer, Reiner Fuellmich, would account for the dualistic thinking, primal emotional reactions, cruelty, and other personality changes observed in the vaccinated.

"This has been a war on the human and what makes us human," Wolf observed, "and if an injection can close down people's compassion or their higher powers of nuanced critical thinking, it could close down their connection to a sense of spirituality. It could close down their sense of responsibility to the next generation. We don't know. This is a mass experiment on the human brain and the human heart."

Also on the call was Peter Breggin, a renowned psychiatrist known as 'The Conscience of Psychiatry' for putting a stop to lobotomies and other atrocities in U.S. psychiatry. The vaccine's effect on the brain, he said, was similar to that of lobotomy and electroshock treatment where, in a hierarchy of losses, "The first loss is love," along with the most complex, subtle, and finely tuned human attributes of affiliation, caring, and moral restraint. "It just reduces the ability of the soul to communicate through the brain."

Social engineering is in play, Breggin infers, because "The frontal lobes contain our civilization." The vaccine agenda sought to bring about a listless, compliant population that could be more easily controlled. because there are "too many problem people… What is better for totalitarian mass than producing docility, lack of being able to plan anything like a rebellion?"

Food scientist, Mike Adams, draws similar conclusions. In an October 2023 broadcast, he warned, "We're talking about slow-acting lobotomies that are taking down the cognitive function of much of America."

Mere genocide, then, did not satisfy the murderous appetites of Pfizer and the infernal deities it serves. It also stole into human consciousness, defiled its sacred temples, usurped its holy throne. Pfizer's mission was not just to kill the perishable body but to torture the imperishable soul.

CONCLUSION

20 QUESTIONS FOR PFIZER

Parsing truth from lies in Pfizer's Biological Product File was a huge labour. By now, the released documents number hundreds of thousands of pages. But I am glad to have helped demolish that Satanic temple known as Pfizer. Below are 20 questions to close out this series.

1/ Why did Pfizer start recruiting clinical-trial investigators in 2018?

Two PDF documents (Part A and Part B) contain CVs (resumés) of some 160 investigators who conducted clinical trials for Pfizer's serum in six countries. Three CVs are signed in 2018, 10 in 2019, and 14 in the first quarter of 2020. Why so many recruits before a so-called 'pandemic' was even declared?

2/ Why did Pfizer include adolescents in clinical trials for its COVID 'vaccine' when it knew this was illegal?

Pfizer began recruiting participants aged 12 through 15 for its adolescent trials in October 2020, but in *AGREED PEDIATRIC STUDY PLAN*, written somewhere between December 2020 and May 2021, Pfizer wrote, "Pfizer and BioNTech propose to request a deferral of the evaluation of the COVID-19 vaccine in individuals ≤15 years of age" (p.8).

To support this request, Pfizer cited the *Pediatric Research Equity Act of 2003* (21 U.S. Code § 355c) which states, "Pediatric studies should be delayed until additional safety or effectiveness data have been collected" (Section 505B (3)(A)). Thus, Pfizer knew what the legislation required and made it clear that it knew, but conducted the trial anyway. Why?

3/ Why did Pfizer refuse to cover the medical bills of a 12-year-old girl paralyzed during the trial?

On Jan. 20, 2021, Maddie de Garay, a healthy and athletic 12-year-old girl, received a second dose in Pfizer's two-dose clinical trial for adolescents at Cincinnati Children's Hospital. About 18 hours later, she developed severe pain throughout her body. Her heart felt like it was being pulled out. Over the following months, she lost the ability to swallow food or liquids, and had to resort to a feeding tube. She experienced fainting spells which developed into seizures, sometimes 10 a day. Finally, she lost feeling from the waist down, which led to paralysis and incontinence.

But lead trial investigator, Dr. Robert Frenck, told Maddie's parents in a May 17, 2021 phone call that they were solely responsible for covering Maddie's medical bills at Cincinnati Children's.

As stated in the *Declaration of Helsinki—Ethical Principles for Medical Research Involving Human Subjects*, "Appropriate compensation and treatment for subjects who are harmed as a result of participating in research must be ensured" (Para. 15).

Why did Pfizer desecrate this?

4/ Why did Frenck claim Pfizer's 'vaccine' "had a favorable safety and side-effect profile"?

Frenck asserted Pfizer's 'vaccine' "had a favorable safety and side-effect profile" in a May 2021 article reporting on the adolescents trial in which Maddie participated. Published in *The New England Journal of Medicine* (*NEJM*), the article also claimed, "there were no vaccine-related serious adverse events and few overall severe adverse events" (p.1). Why did NEJM publish Frenck's lies? Why did neither Pfizer nor the FDA rein him in?

5/ Why did Pfizer enlist Frenck to run another vaccine trial in 2021?

Frenck led another study at Cincinnati Children's Hospital from February 2021 to July 2021, this time into 'lot consistency' (Protocol C4591017). One participant in the trial experienced a spontaneous abortion, though Frenck deemed this was unrelated to the study vaccine. Why did Pfizer rehire this obviously corrupt investigator? (The study report redacts the lead investigator's name, but I have confirmed it was Frenck.)

6/ Why did Frenck's lot-consistency study run with only four manufacturing lots when it was originally designed to examine five?

The study tested three lots from the U.S. and one from Europe though, according to a March 2021 paper published in *Springer Nature,* five lots were originally intended. Who changed the parameters, and why?

7/ Why did the lot-consistency study conceal the lot numbers tested?

Vast differences have been observed in the lethality and harm of Pfizer shots according to their batch numbers, and there are thousands of those numbers. Pfizer's first *Periodic Safety Update Report* (*PSUR #1*) to the European Medicines Agency (EMA) listed 19 lot numbers associated with the highest numbers of adverse events.

But the lot-consistency study does not mention which lot numbers were tested, listing them only as 'US Lot 1', 'US Lot 2', etc., so that correlation is impossible. What were the lot numbers used?

8/ Where did the 29 fatalities happen during clinical trials for Pfizer's booster? And where are the autopsy results?

In its third *Periodic Safety Update Report (PSUR #3)* to the EMA (reporting period Dec. 19, 2021 to June 18, 2022), Pfizer tallies 29 fatal outcomes in clinical trials for its booster (p.81). How are those fatalities split among the trials listed (C4591001, C4591031, C4591024, C4591007, BNT162-17, and C4591030)? (The youngest recipient of a booster in these trials was 1.4 years.)

Also, as Pfizer's *Dose-Finding Study* document stipulates several times, "In the case of a participant death, a summary of available autopsy findings must be submitted as soon as possible to Pfizer Safety" (e.g., p.110). Were those findings gathered? If so, where are they?

9/ What happened to hundreds of missing babies?

Pfizer notes, in its 'Analysis of Booster Doses' in *PSUR #3,* that 455 babies who experienced adverse events during the six-month period were excluded from the analysis "due to indirect exposure (transplacental/transmammary) to BNT162b2," meaning they were affected in the womb and/or at the breast from an injected mother (p.80). What were the individual outcomes for each of those 455?

10/ What happened to Pfizer's plan to inject newborns?

Another biological product-file document, *License Action Recommendation Documents for Submissions and FDA Communication,* shows Pfizer was talking with the FDA in July 2021 about "another study to enroll infants <6 months of age" (p.10). When and why were those plans shelved?

11/ Who "injected with force"?

PSUR #3 tallies a litany of 'Medication Errors' that befell 68,025 jab recipients in its six-month reporting period alone. One of these was "injected with force" (p.106). What were the circumstances of this incident? There were also seven cases where "The subject intentionally refused to be vaccinated or was not able to receive the scheduled BNT162b2." Was coercion used or attempted?

12/ Why did Pfizer's investigator cover up pericarditis injury?

As spotted by scientist and author, Dr. David Healy,

troubling anomalies appear in the clinical-trial results Pfizer put in its Biological Product File. One example is a 66-year-old man, with no reported medical history, who enrolled in Pfizer's COVID-vaccine (C4591001) trial in Buenos Aires (subject number 12315632).

On Oct. 18, 2020, the man was hospitalized with chest pain and shortness of breath, 29 days after receiving a second Pfizer injection, and diagnosed with pericarditis (*16.2.7.1 Adverse Events,* p.3,367). But, in another document, the recorded diagnosis for the same individual is "suspected COVID-19," though he tested negative for SARS-CoV-2 three times (p.997). The pericarditis isn't even mentioned.

13/ Why did Pfizer's trial in pregnant women (C4591015) limit its scope to third-trimester pregnancies?

According to the March 2021 paper in *Springer Nature,* Pfizer planned to trial its vaccine in healthy pregnant women, aged 18 and older, at 24 to 34 weeks' gestation (C4591015/ NCT04713553). Why, when health authorities have urged and cajoled pregnant women to get COVID jabs at every stage of gestation, was this limitation applied for the trial?

14/ Where are the results for pregnant women?

Pfizer's study on pregnant women (C4591015) ran

from Feb. 16, 2021 to July 15, 2022, but it has still not released. the results. When will they be released?

15/ Do any Pfizer COVID injections contain luciferase?

In developing its COVID injection, Pfizer used the firefly enzyme, luciferase, in 'biodistribution' studies on rats and mice. It was used to observe where injection components would end up by seeing which body parts glowed with 'bioluminescence'. Moderna lists luciferase as a component of its own COVID vaccine in patent US 10,703,789 (p.46, Table 4). Is luciferase also in the 'vaccine' Pfizer rolled out to the public?

16/ Do any Pfizer COVID injections contain graphene or graphene oxide?

Graphene oxide is lethally toxic to humans, destroying cells and damaging DNA. We know it is used in Pfizer's manufacturing process from a paper in Pfizer's Biological Product File. How much graphene oxide is making its way into Pfizer's serums and thence into the human body?

17/ Spike protein. Where's the off-switch?

Spike proteins are extremely toxic to the human body and, as has been known since at least 2007, cause cell injury and cell death. They also cross the blood-brain barrier and permeate other organs of the body. Yet Pfizer designed its COVID injections to have the human body produce more of them, which in turn risks further harm from autoimmune attack. What mechanism is included in the shots to turn off spike-protein production?

18/ Will Pfizer abandon mRNA 'therapies'?

In its SEC filing for 2020, Pfizer acknowledged, "mRNA therapies have been classified as gene therapy medicinal products… Any product candidates we develop may not be effective, may be only moderately effective, or may prove to have undesirable or unintended side effects, toxicities or other characteristics that may preclude our obtaining marketing approval or prevent or limit commercial use."

Given overwhelming evidence that mRNA therapies do cause toxicity and harm—far surpassing all previous vaccines—will Pfizer now abandon this destructive technology?

19/ Why is simian virus in the Pfizer shot?

Professor Murukami, of the Tokyo University of Science, has found Pfizer shots contain simian virus 40 (SV40) which, according to a 2004 paper, "induces primary brain and bone cancers, malignant mesothelioma, and lymphomas in laboratory animals." What is it doing in Pfizer's COVID medicine?

20/ Why did Pfizer turn the penis into a bioweapon?

In its consent form for clinical trials, dated July 2020, Pfizer told participants, "Men may not donate sperm until 60 days after the last vaccination." Why did women, and potential offspring, need protection from the sperm of injected men?

INTRODUCTION TO 'KNOW YOUR MEDICAL RIGHTS'

BOOK 1 IN 'BATTLE MANUALS FOR FREEEDOM

I was brought up by my mother on the Bible, and she told me something that I've never forgotten. She said the stories in the Bible are stories about the conflict between the kings who have power and the prophets who preach righteousness, and she taught me to support the prophets and not the kings.

— TONY BENN, FORMER BRITISH MEMBER OF PARLIAMENT, MAR. 10, 2006

I am writing this book because I have to, and because I know a confrontation is coming. No longer can I maintain the old uneasy coexistence with false authority, lamenting his folly and fraud, deploring his ignorance, and ridiculing his absurdities, but all from a safe distance. No, I am on a collision course with false authority, and I dare say you are too. We need to be prepared.

I have lived and worked on four continents, swum in

three oceans, heard innumerable foreign tongues, and observed the infinite variety of our species, but now the autocrats, bureaucrats, and technocrats, in their little, brief, and fear-fueled authority, would have us undergo invasive medical procedures, and hand over private medical information once held sacred, just to travel, to go about our lives, and even to make a living.

Time was when I could grudgingly accept mask requirements in the early days, frown at destructive lockdowns, and ignore voicemails and messages to my mobile phone from Britain's National Health Service (NHS). And I could largely dismiss the barrage of fearmongering propaganda that managed to circumvent my longstanding aversion to mainstream media. But when governments started threatening and penalizing bodily autonomy, a line was crossed.

I know in my heart that these measures are an atrocity, and my spirit rebels against them, but just having that instinct is not enough now. **WHAT ARE MY RIGHTS?!** I'm going to need more than mere disgust if I am to overrule the fearmongering autocrats who will exploit any emergency to unleash tyranny. I'm going to need constitutional armour and weapons of law, and I'm going to need them quickly. And when I have them, I will share them with those who may benefit.

Hence this book, a garment of protection for the 'COVID' era and an antidote to fear. I don't mean fear of a disease, but of the reactions—or rather overreactions—to it. Though I once entertained some background anxiety about a supposed virus, it's as nothing compared to the deep dread I've experienced about a totalitarian state emerging such as Orwell set out in *1984*.

I have also come to realize that even *that* kind of fear is being stoked by governments. At the outset, they wanted us to fear COVID, but after that got them only so far, now they want us to fear them, so that we won't make trouble.

For that type of fear, I recall the predicament of Moses' Israelites lately released from slavery in Egypt, as recounted in the Bible book of *Exodus*. Imagine their terror to realize Pharaoh's entire army was bearing down on them as they approached the Red Sea (14:10). But Moses told them not to fear, to stand firm, for they would see the Lord's deliverance. And they did, when the Red Sea drowned Pharaoh and his horde (14:28).

Therefore, no matter how bad things appear to get, the final chapter of our story sees the demise of slavery on Earth, including wage slavery, debt slavery, tax slavery, prison slavery, sex slavery, digital slavery and, of course, medical slavery, along with the deaths of tyrant politicians, bureaucrats, and corporate profiteers when, like a mighty river, Justice returns.

The 'vaccines', too, have an obvious allegory in the *Exodus* story. When Moses and his brother Aaron come to Pharaoh's court and issue their demands, Aaron demonstrates the power of God by turning his staff into a snake. Pharaoh's conjurors imitate the act, but Aaron's snake eats their snakes (7:12). Similarly, the fanged creatures of Pfizer, Moderna, AstraZeneca, and Johnson &

Johnson are no match for the lethal bite of truth-tellers, prophets, and whistleblowers today.

Also destined for destruction are the media organizations who have mouthpieced for the medical-industrial complex. I shudder to recall the *Daily Telegraph* front-page headline of July 21, 2021: "Freedom for double jabbed as UK opens to world." As if freedom can be granted or withheld at official whim, as if medical status were the qualification to receive it. No, we are born with it, and trying to take it away from us is blasphemy, no less an atrocity than the 'intercision' of Philip Pullman's novel, *The Golden Compass,* where the authorities cut children away from their 'daemon' animals, equivalent to extracting their souls.

The *Telegraph* also predicted, in a July-2021 article, "The unvaccinated will be shut out of normal life, progressively demonised, and stripped of civil rights..." And other mainstream outlets salivated at the prospect. As 2021 drew to a close, a quick glance at recent headlines showed an almost desperate eagerness to foment hatred against a vilified underclass. "The unvaccinated are putting us all at risk," squealed *The Times* of London. "I'm Furious at the Unvaccinated," howled *The New York Times*. "It is only a matter of time before we turn on the unvaccinated," thundered *The Guardian*.

Just like the cultist politicians and bureaucrats, these media mercenaries for Big Pharma know not what they say or what they do. Nor do they know or care that international statute defines persecution against an identifiable group as a Crime Against Humanity. Have all these puppets learned nothing from history and the madness of going after a targeted minority? Has it taken but a few generations to overturn what our ancestors fought and died for? Have these people lost their minds? I think they have!

We of prophetic calling have our work cut out for us, not just seeing, or warning against, future scenarios, as exemplified by Orwell, but in describing the present. That means observing the obvious and stating the obvious when populations are conditioned to overlook the obvious, to deny it to themselves and, even if they do see it, to keep quiet about it. As famed whistleblower Edward Snowden observes, "Everywhere we look, from Afghanistan to economics, from pandemic to pervasive surveillance, the obvious has been made unspeakable."[i]

And it is obvious that the medical-industrial complex, taking its playbook from the *military*-industrial complex, grooms politicians to do its bidding. It also likens the COVID response to war, reflecting the imperial and imperious mindset infecting our politics, with words like battle, beat, conquer, crush, defeat, eliminate, enemy, fight, front lines, victory, etc.

There *is* a war being waged, certainly, but of a very different kind, as encapsulated by the apostle Paul in the New Testament: "For our struggle is not against flesh and blood, but against the rulers, against the authorities, against the powers of this dark world and against the spiritual forces of evil in the heavenly realms" (*Ephesians* 6:12).

And those spiritual forces are especially murderous

towards children, recalling the ancient abomination of child sacrifice to Molech.

> "The Lord said to Moses, 'Say to the Israelites: Any Israelite or any foreigner residing in Israel who sacrifices any of his children to Molek is to be put to death. The members of the community are to stone him. I myself will set my face against him and will cut him off from his people; for by sacrificing his children to Molek, he has defiled my sanctuary and profaned my holy name. If the members of the community close their eyes when that man sacrifices one of his children to Molek and if they fail to put him to death, I myself will set my face against him and his family and will cut them off from their people, together with all who follow him in prostituting themselves to Molek.' "
>
> — *LEVITICUS* 20:1-5

Of course, fraud, corruption, and greed have always greased the wheels of government, but now we observe something far deadlier, a medical cult that demands human sacrifice, a religion of death, served by a conclave of tyrant priests in positions of false authority. The more they can kill, the higher they rise in their infernal ranks.

I wish the figureheads of our so-called 'medical-freedom movement' would see this. I wish they would realize that the pharmaceutical complex is not so much counting the dollars as it is counting the bodies.

I came to this realization when hearing renowned

liver-health specialist and author, Dr. Burt Berkson, tell Dr. Jonathan Landsman in an interview, "At many medical schools, in many university hospitals, they give an award every month to the doctor who has the most deaths on his service, and they have a party, and it's called a 'Black Crow Award'."

Is that what this is all about? Are we in the middle of a global Black Crow Award now, in which medical professionals and hospitals and so-called health ministers are competing to see who can add the most corpses to the pile of medical waste? Or have they been assigned kill quotas?

That medical-freedom leaders overlook this deeper motivation is disappointing, but many more errors, and possibly fatal ones, they make besides. Most dangerous of all is to base their opposition to medical compulsion not on the solid ground that it is eternally unlawful, but on the shifting sands of data and statistics.

For example, they argue that this disease, or that variant, is too mild to warrant medical enforcements. Meaning what? That if some more deadly disease were conjured, they'd be fine with coercion?

That is boggy ground to build on, to paraphrase Herman Melville. Of course, autocrats are always ready to unleash another emergency which they will cite as pretext for more crackdowns and despotic legislation that they falsely call 'law'.

We also hear the medical-freedom caucus arguing certain measures should not be mandated because they are unproven, unsafe, or ineffective. Or because natural immunity is a thing, or asymptomatic spread is not a thing.

Fools! There is no 'because'! No medical measure can ever be compulsory—period, end of—whatever claims are asserted for its safety or effectiveness.

And here's the stupidest slogan of all. "Where there is risk, there must be choice." Meaning what? That if some medical treatment is concocted, and safety claimed for it, then choice can be taken away?

Misguided, too, are requests for 'exemption' from medical enforcement. These buy into a fiction that government has authority to demand anything from us in the first place. It doesn't. Quite the opposite. We have authority over government, and the word "No" is, always has been, and always will be, exemption enough.

Exemption requests also desecrate medical confidentiality when your medical status is nobody else's business in the first place. It is not the government's business, not your employer's business, not a travel company's business, and not your neighbour's business. Respect confidentiality, and your medical status can never be weaponized against you.

Our resolve against medical dictatorship, therefore, can never rest on competing views about today's data and circumstances but must instead be anchored in **CONSTITUTIONALITY**. Blind to emergency by design, constitutional principles are eternal and can't be swayed by the shifting currents of perception and statistics. They don't give a fuck about conditions on the ground, and nor should they. No, these times call us to be **CONSTITUTIONAL EXTREMISTS**.

Lawyers, too, need to grasp this. They whimper about not being able to go after pharmaceutical companies, doctors, hospitals, or regulators because of 'legal immunity'. Servile creatures, I rebuke your compliance with tyrant fictions spun to enslave Mankind. The Acts and statutes you cite—and stop calling them laws—these licences to kill, are nothing more than corporate contracts that one party has drafted, one party has signed, and one party has negotiated with itself. Yet that party thinks to impose those contracts on another party, us, to codify enslavement, murder, extortion, destruction, and theft, and then to pardon itself of the crimes. As we shall see, in the coming section on Common Law, these instruments are powerless without our signature, and not worth the air they're written on.

Imagine you were a business owner seeking to procure goods from a supplier, but that supplier gets to write the contract without your review, and that contract binds you as soon as the ink is dry without your knowledge, signature, or consent. You'd tell them to get lost, wouldn't you? Yet that is precisely the bargain that governments and their corporate conspirators think to impose, and before which our conditioned cadre of cringing lawyers think to kneel. When will you stop enthroning legislation over Justice?!

One rare exception to this tendency is British human-rights lawyer, Anna de Buisseret. Interviewed in London's

Parliament Square during a Medical Freedom March of Oct. 30, 2021, she advises:

> "Learn what your fundamental, inalienable human rights are. Anyone who can access Google, you google the Universal Declaration of Human Rights, read it, read the European Convention on Human Rights, read the U.K. Human Rights Act, read the International Covenant on Social and Political and Economic Rights. Those rights are all there. It's all there in the law. The reason this is happening is because people don't know the law, so they don't know how to uphold it and assert it."

I applaud the spirit of her words, though that's an awful lot of homework for your average freedom-loving reader to do, especially if you add in the 170-page Notice of Liability, prepared by de Buisseret and her allies in Lawyers for Liberty, to serve against skin piercers and their accomplices. But I *have* done the homework and distilled into this book the key language that empowers us.

The good news is that none of this is complicated. It doesn't require a law degree, nor a thorough grounding in Latin. The beauty of these universal principles lies in their plain-English simplicity and, like the proverbial mustard seed of faith that overthrows mountains,[ii] our little understanding in this arena goes a long way in vaulting the pronouncements of foolish and fearful men. A layman's expertise will do, and a layman's analysis can provide it, which is why I am as qualified as anyone else to do so here.

Brothers and sisters, it is time to release from their glass cabinets the dusty scrolls of our Rights declarations. We reclaim the keys that unleash them and, like the true prophets of old, proclaim them again to break the spells and incantations of false priests now roaming the Earth.

Our Rights, being inalienable, or unalienable if you prefer, were never granted by a gift of government nor rescinded by a denial of government. In the words of John K. Webster, creator of the documentary *Strawman*,

> **"GOVERNMENT IS A CREATION OF MAN, AND A CREATION OF MAN CAN NEVER BE ABOVE MAN."**

So, if governments will not hear or heed the simple and time-honoured constitutional principles they are sworn to uphold, then each of us must acquire at least a little expertise in this area.

Nor will I pin my hopes on a political party or candidate to produce a regime a little less vindictive than the last. Love for our Rights straddles the old divides where antagonists are merely co-conspirators in bipartisan acts of theft. As Martin Luther wrote of the papists and anabaptists in 1531, "These foxes are tied together by the tails, even though their heads look in opposite directions. While they outwardly profess to be great enemies, inwardly they think, teach, and defend one and the same thing." Once we realize this, and expose the unholy alliances against our core values, whether by Democrat with Republican, Tory with Labour, or by any other duopoly or coalition, we can be rid of this corrupt political theatre altogether.

We are in a Declaration-of-Independence moment when an entire *form* of government, not just a faction *within* government, is destroying Life, Liberty, and the Pursuit of Happiness. It is therefore our duty now to abolish *this* form of government, maybe even the entire *idea* of government (which means 'mind control'). We are not fighting in a horizontal plane of 'Left' versus 'Right', but in the vertical plane of Life over Death, Creation over Destruction, Love over Fear.

That is a spiritual battle, the battle for which this book is conceived. May this declaration in words empower us to "suit the action to the word, the word to the action"[iii] as we hear and heed the rallying call from the Captain of our souls, he whose Word "is alive and active, and sharper than any double-edged sword" (*Hebrews* 4:12).

Allied with that weapon is our sword of constitutional truth. It pulses with Heaven's call for Justice, imparts courage to those who wield it, and thirsts for the blood of today's cabal of thieves and murderers, whether in government, media, or any other organization. Let us pursue them with the kind of fury that Elijah wielded in slaughtering the false prophets of Baal on Mount Carmel (*1 Kings* 18:40). For, as Dave Mason writes in his masterful *Age of Prophecy* novels,[iv] set in the time of Elijah,

"Those who show mercy to the cruel, bring cruelty upon the merciful."

For those of us contemplating our first run-in with would-be enforcers such as police, the task ahead may appear daunting, but here I share the vital information we will need if menaced by state or corporation, and if you have a paperback version, I hope it shall become marked up with your highlights and scribblings. Our quest may seem to present impossible odds. Well, you would have said the same of Moses and Aaron going up against Pharaoh, his court, his paymasters, slave masters, chariots, and weaponry. But he who was in the prophets was greater than he who was in Pharaoh, and he who is in us now is greater than he who is in the autocrats, bureaucrats, technocrats, and 'psychocrats' of our age. And, oh yes, the 'philanthrocrats' too!

"Hold the line, stand your ground, uphold the rule of law, step into your sovereignty," De Buisseret urges in the closing moments of her Parliament-Square interview. "The law is all there to protect you, but you're not going to get protected unless you know what it is and you uphold it."

Therefore, we look to the eternal values of Mankind—values not swayed by political convenience and expediency, nor by profiteering motives, and that have *more* currency, not less, during times of emergency, whether that emergency is real or perceived or invented. So join me in the field, my friend. These times will make prophets of us all!

INTRODUCTION TO 'KNOW YOUR LAWFUL RIGHTS'

BOOK 2 IN 'BATTLE MANUALS FOR FREEDOM'

> *The elite's goal is disturbingly straightforward: to hollow out the individual, leaving an empty shell while stripping away the soul.*
>
> — A LILY BIT, *THE EXPOSE*, MAR. 15, 2024

We were born into slavery, but until recently, most of us did not know it. With subtle treachery, banks, corporations, and governments have stolen our Birthright. Spiritual vampires, they have drained us of our time and energies, even of life itself, to enrich themselves. It took the atrocities of COVID to alert us to this, to shake us awake, and to break the spell that has been perpetrated against Mankind for centuries and even millennia.

Some were aware of the tyrants' genocidal plans even

before COVID, and for that you have my deepest respect. You did your best to warn everyone what evil was afoot, and you saved lives. Though you were censored and reviled, you stuck to your message, and then I joined you to expose how broad and deep is the conspiracy against us. In early 2022, I published *The COVID Protocols: Upholding Your Rights in Authoritarian Times,* now retitled *Know Your Medical Rights*. I thought this would be enough, but when the despotism spread from the medical arena to every other area of life, I realized COVID was just the first round in a barrage of assaults aimed at demolishing our lives, our livelihoods, and all that makes life worth living. I would need to write more books.

I agree with Dr. Rima Laibow's observation, in a March 2024 interview with Maria Zeee, that…

> "There is no aspect of human life which will be allowed to continue as we know it, as we value it. And most of all, what is being destroyed is the capacity to love and to trust one another. So we are being separated from our wisdom, from our bodies, from our DNA, from our children, from our property, from our very capacity to bring food forth from the Earth. We are being separated from our ability to think, to communicate, all of it in the interest of a vast and total suppression of humanity into a slave caste that can never rise up again. To which my response is, 'No! Out! I want out of your system!' "

Yes, Dr. Rima has poetically described the breadth of tyranny now afoot, but I am astonished too by its depth.

It starts with international puppet masters, usually described as 'globalists', who take their orders from secret societies and the infernal influences that inspire them. Then, the tyranny is channeled through their network of despots installed in national governments and other corporations.

The infestation doesn't stop there, though, for regional and local governments, county councils, town councils, planning departments, and even school boards and housing associations are fully on board with the despotic agenda of enslavement and destruction, either as complicit operatives or as useful idiots.

Police forces, meanwhile, corporate henchmen and bandits for hire, are enforcing all of this. How refreshing it would be if just one stood up and said, "No sir. That's an unlawful order." What a revelation if just one upheld their Oath. Instead, we are treated to the shameful spectacle of police beating up, trampling, and irradiating protesters, menacing journalists, arresting people for praying in public, and even issuing tickets against those who feed the homeless. And that's just what they do in public. Meanwhile, they give protective escort to today's agents of doom when angry crowds come too close.

COVID also taught me a new word: democide, defined in the *Collins Dictionary* as "the killing of members of a country's civilian population as a result of its government's policy, including by direct action, indifference, and neglect." I now realize that governments of the West have been doing this for decades, but they got much more unsubtle and extreme about it with COVID, both with the murderous protocols deployed in hospitals and nursing homes, then with the coerced poison injections they called 'vaccines'. Since then, among many vectors of attack, they have gone after our food, our fuel, and funds too.

I laugh when I hear people talk about "government overreach" or when they say, "The government doesn't have your best interests at heart." OK, I suppose you could call genocide 'overreach', but strip away the varnish and you will see a regime that wants to enslave you, to extract every ounce of value it can from your life and labour then, when you've nothing left to give, to discard you as cheaply as possible and add your corpse to the growing pile of medical waste. And if that's too much of a mouthful, your government simply wants to kill you!

Nor are legislators doing much to check rogue administrations. As 'Health Ranger' Mike Adams said in a May 2024 broadcast,...

> "All they do every single day in the halls of Congress is they figure out, 'How can we hurt America today? How do we harm the American people? How do we vote against the interests of the American people?' They're straight-up traitors. Every single day, they conspire of how to destroy this country from within."

And that conspiracy is entirely 'legal' in the sense that politicians, or rather their handlers, have drawn up documents that not only codify their thefts and murders but shield them from consequence with so-called 'legal immunity'. I tend to agree with Max Igan's encapsulation, in a February 2024 broadcast, that "Every single problem on Earth exists because it has been legislated to exist."

Which brings me to a central theme of this book, and that is to draw a clear distinction between 'legal' and 'lawful', for they are very different things and usually contrary. 'Legal' pertains to the legislation that men create—Acts, statutes, rules, regulations, decrees, and codes, the injustice of which corporate courts cement with their rulings. 'Lawful', by contrast, belongs only to the Creator, whom to serve is Freedom (*John* 8:36; 2 *Corinthians* 3:17) and whose burden is light (*Matthew* 11:28-30), and it respects our inherent Rights and dignity. These Rights may be enshrined in constitutions but they don't depend on constitutions for their existence or applicability.

As Living Men and Women operating in the Lawful, which is our Birthright, we are wholly above the Legal. Indeed, as three-dimensional beings, we are an entire *dimension* above the Legal, which operates only in the two-dimensional realm of words on paper. Those words cannot reach up from the page, grab us by the neck, and pull us down into their flattened space, though that is what their devisers intend. No, those documents are dead to us, and we refuse to breathe life into them by consenting to them with our signatures. In the three-dimensional realm where we live and move and breathe and have our beings, Government cannot even touch us, much less dictate to us.

Yet politicians, along with enforcers and

commentators, routinely ascribe to tyrant code the false label of 'Law'. It's all fiction, all counterfeit. By True Law, or 'Common Law', those who deliberately do harm must face Justice, while the falsely accused are innocent if there is no victim.

More troubling still, the fallacy of calling rules made up by men and women 'Law' is echoed by so-called alternative voices, Freedom warriors, and 'truthers' who should know better. This one error has me "shouting at the radio" more than any other.

For example, Katherine Watt, whose work I respect, routinely makes the mistake of calling legislation 'Law', so does Sasha Latypova. I have heard James Delingpole, Catherine Austin Fitts, Peggy Hall, Greg Reese, James Roguski, Jane Ruby, Scott Schara, and Maria Zeee all err on this point. Mike Adams makes this error in almost every episode of his Health Ranger Report, and Todd Callender in almost every sentence.

I respect their research, but through this one abuse of language alone, they unwittingly confer on governments a false authority to play God in the lives of others; dictate to us what we must do with our bodies, our property, our children, and even out thoughts; and then have us bend the knee and plead for 'exemptions' that they may grant at their pleasure by a counterfeit mercy.

Lawyers, too, are generally taking government writ as gospel by confining their range of motion to the shrinking legal box of legislation. Even to call them 'lawyers' is a misnomer when, for the most part, they are not dealing in Law at all but in the muck of legislation. They are not lawyers but corporate power-brokers and negotiators cutting deals with corporate entities, wherein you and I are regarded as no more than corporations.

So, if there's only one thing you take away from this book, let it be this...

STOP CALLING LEGISLATION LAW!

This one shift in mindset will produce good fruit. You will see legislation for the toilet fodder it really is, and even 'legislation' may be too generous a term because the entities that forge it, pretend to debate it, and dutifully pass it are all corporations, that is to say, invented things, and their prolixious documents amount to nothing more than corporate policy, binding only upon themselves and their own employees. All governments, parliaments, courts, and police forces *are* corporations, and their policies, procedures, and decrees have no more authority over us than if McDonald's or Starbucks had written them.

It boils down to this: God makes Law, man makes legislation, and corporations make company policy. How dare they ascribe to men and to the institutions of men the authority to make Law? When there is already so little airtime afforded genuine voices for Freedom, we cannot afford to build on such a broken foundation.

Further, Acts and statutes are, in effect, contracts that one party draws up, one party negotiates with itself, and one party signs, and then thinks to impose on another party, us, without our signature or consent, much less our

Informed Consent. Governments and corporations may not impose any demand on you unless you have voluntarily, and with full knowledge, signed a contract that includes your agreement to the demand. Therefore, if some would-be enforcer tells you, "You have to do this. This is the law," you say, "Show me the document that says this, and show me where I signed it."

Still, I wrestled with calling this book, *Know Your Legal Rights* instead of *Know Your Lawful Rights*. Though the Lawful is as far above the Legal as the heavens are above the Earth, we may on occasion operate in the Legal, and though we are not subject to the pieces of paper written by men, we may still cite them on a Legal stage to compel enforcers to obey the contracts binding upon themselves.

If we enter the Legal, therefore, we do so as an actor puts on a costume to play a role. We do not *live* in the Legal, any more than an actor would live his entire life in the costume and lines of his character, but we may play a role in it sometimes. Imagine the hell of an actor trapped forever in the fictional time and place of his theatrical persona with no way out, even worse if he lost all memory of his prior life outside the role and forgot there was an exit. That nightmarish condition describes much of Humanity today, but not you or me. If we ever operate in the Legal, we remember that we are not *of* the Legal.

In the end, I went with *Lawful* for the title, because that is the realm of Truth, whereas Legal is the realm of fiction. Like a thieving usurper, Legal has crept into the throne room of our Sovereignty and presumes to rule as

King, but he is an impostor and must be ousted if we are to restore our Birthright in the Lawful.

This requires a shift in mindset. We have much to learn, or rather unlearn, as we dismantle the lies, programming, and conditioning that have kept us from ourselves. The walls of my own perception too must dissolve to write this book. Ironically, COVID did much of that work for me by exposing the evil, and the doers of that evil, that have long crouched in the shadows and quietly infested our institutions. As the poet Theodore Roethke wrote, "In a dark time the eye begins to see." I imagine God's hand on the dimmer switch of our awareness and gradually turning up the light.

And as that dawn returns, Government shall no longer be enthroned in the minds of men, nor shall its ideologies, stupidity, or stupid ideologies. Alas, the evildoers have been assisted in their acts of theft and destruction by a largely compliant population. People seem to have embedded in their consciousness, "I must obey Government," turning it into a religion. Even after the COVID era, with its ample demonstration that Government is a cult seeking our enslavement and death, this idea is still firmly lodged in most people.

For example, I notice when taking flights in the U.S. that I am the only one refusing the body-scan chambers that the Transport and Security Administration (TSA) puts people through, the photos taken after international arrivals, and the biometric scans even at departure gates, all of which are Fourth-Amendment violations and, in the case of the body scans, medical violations too. Seeing the compliance of others is deeply frightening to me because they will passively watch tyranny happen to others and just stand idly by, or perhaps get out their mobile phones to record it and win coveted clicks on social media. At their worst, they will turn in their neighbours, or even other family members, and report non-compliance to the authorities.

I also recently saw a New Zealand honey producer torching his hives and with them, millions of bees, because the government told him to. Before that, an Australian producer allowed government agents on to his property where they drowned his bees in petrol. It is an enraging spectacle. The bees, at least, have enough regard for their own survival to sting their attackers, but many compliant humans have no sting of their own, even when directly assailed.

In Britain, meanwhile, households keeping even a single chicken are "required" to register their bird. To anyone paying even perfunctory attention, it is obvious the government will at some point try to use this information to destroy every last vestige of independent food production by conjuring some disease scare such as 'bird flu' and culling yet more hens.

Why do people keep falling for these deceptions? I want to shake them and say, "Moron, the government is trying to destroy you and your business, and the food supply along with it!" And if the autocrats can't entirely cause starvation, they are doing their best to destroy independent farmers who might produce clean, healthy food. That way, they can force consumption of their highly processed, poison-laced megacorporation stomach fillers sold in supermarkets which, in turn, are extremely vulnerable to supply-line sabotage.

Even the very word, 'Government'—which means 'mind control'—is offensive to me now. Who do these people think they are to 'govern' anyone, let alone to tax us, especially when they operate in, and are promoted by, a system that rewards corruption, laziness, and incompetence, in a culture of failing upwards? As Christ said of the Pharisees in his day, "they bind heavy burdens and grievous to be borne, and lay them on men's shoulders, but do not lift a finger to help them" (*Matthew* 23:4).

In Jesus' day, the Pharisees were a hypocritical religious cult, whitewashed tombs full of dead men's bones as he described them, a brood of vipers who strain out gnats but swallow camels (*Matthew* 23). Similarly, today's Pharisees strain out gnats by punishing speech that offends them while swallowing camels of rape, genocide, and theft. Meanwhile, their religion demands of us extortionate tithes, offerings, sacrifices, and ritual performances as, almost every day, they issue some new decree to control us, some new fine or some new fee, and then expect us dutifully to follow and to obey, to follow and to pay.

In the process, our constitutions and Rights declarations are routinely trampled in the name of virtue-signalling slogans such as 'diversity', 'equity', 'inclusion', 'prevention', 'safety', 'security', 'sustainability', and so on. These are empty words when they come from the mouths of tyrants and, as Homer reminds us in *The Odyssey*, "Empty words are evil" (XI.544).

We must therefore reclaim our inherent authority and remember the obvious and irrefutable truth, as stated in the documentary *Strawman*, that "Government is a creation of Man, and a creation of Man can never be above Man." You and I have authority over every thing that Government is and every thing that Government creates. That's just the authority of logic, but Christians have the even more potent authority from our Lord and Saviour to "overcome all the power of the enemy" (*Luke* 10:19), and in case you haven't realized it, governments *are* the enemy.

So I try never to forget, should I face official, police officer, or judge, that I have authority over them and that I am the one giving *them* 'lawful orders', not the other way round, and that, like their father the devil, these operatives must flee when resisted (*James* 4:7). With this book, I am giving shape to that resistance, assembling not just our constitutional weapons but, for those who "put on the full armour of God" (*Ephesians* 6:13), our spiritual weapons too.

I will admit the enormity of this task feels daunting sometimes, for the subject is vaster than any one author can encompass. I do not pretend to have all the answers, and some of my analysis may yet be naive. Just untangling the history of how we got here would take several volumes, delving back even to Biblical times, but what I can do is present the conceptual frameworks to reclaim our Rights, dispel the illusions that have tried to imprison us, fortify your heart for the battles and skirmishes ahead, and introduce you to solutions and solvers.

I also want to minimize the cost and dangers of the non-compliance we must embrace if we want to get through this. Your instincts are already telling you not to comply, and you may be willing to sacrifice for the cause, but let us be smart about our non-compliance, disciplined, and prepared. Let us also be open to learning more, and honing our skills, as time passes, for these are early days in clawing back our Sovereignty.

The God Stuff

Now, having got Biblical with you a few times by now, I recall that some readers objected to my Scriptural references in *Know Your Medical Rights*. If that is you, season your skepticism a while and acknowledge that even our enemies are deeply religious and that their destructive influence cannot be otherwise explained. For example, do they lie? Then entertain the possibility that they serve the Father of Lies (*John* 8:44). Do they couch their tyranny in virtue-signalling language? Then ask if they serve he who masquerades as an angel of light (2 *Corinthians* 11:14-15). Do they persecute those who tell the truth and who try to warn others? Then consider if they worship he who accuses the righteous (*Revelation* 12:10). And, are they predatory? Then witness how they take after the devil who "prowls around like a roaring lion looking for someone to devour" (*1 Peter* 5:8).

Ask yourself, too, if the assaults against our bodies—not just from venomous injections but from poisons in our food, water, air, sea, and land—are motivated by a hatred of the Most High in whose image we are made (*Genesis* 1:26-27).

Also, do they act in concert across nations, writing the same legislation, telling the same lies, and issuing the same decrees, all at the same time? Then consider how they must be coordinating in secret, making secret oaths and secret pacts, and that secret oaths are the currency of secret societies such as Freemasonry. Have you observed officials, elected or otherwise, along with doctors, judges, and police, desecrating their public oaths, whether to the Constitution or Oath of Office, Hippocratic Oath, or Constable's Oath? Could that mean they are instead cleaving to secret oaths? Would you describe them as psychopaths, meaning they can kill, loot, steal, and destroy others, including children, without remorse? Then is it possible their consciences have been seared (*1 Timothy* 4:1-2) during initiation rites of atrocity? You and I have empathy enough to imagine ourselves in someone else's shoes if they tell us we are causing them harm, but that mechanism has been annihilated in the politicians and bureaucrats of today.

And if you are disposed to excuse the naive ranks of secret-society orders, where the higher-ups—or rather, the lower-downs of an inverted pyramid—conceal the real agenda from initiates, know that even at the First Degree of Freemasonry, they have already condemned themselves by an oath of atrocity. As reported at evangelicaltruth.com, the initiate swears to secrecy "under no less a penalty than that of having my throat cut across, my tongue torn out by its roots, and buried in the rough sands of the sea at low-water mark."

Therefore, show me a Freemason who purports to be a Christian, and I will show you a child of Hell. Christ warned us that no-one can serve two masters, for he will love one and despise the other (*Matthew* 6:24). We infer that the Hell-spawn of today are not just ignoring their public oaths but actively hating them, and that they hate the *Bill of Rights, Magna Carta,* and every other righteous text. Christ also warned that these traitors would plead their good works to him at the Judgment, to which he will reply, "Away from me. I never knew thee!" (*Matthew* 7:22-23).

Meanwhile, you may observe how governments are serving dogmas that try to turn reality upside-down, even going beyond Orwell's "War is peace. Freedom is slavery. Ignorance is strength." In their worldview, good is evil and evil good, love is hate and hate love, health is sickness and sickness health, male is female and female male, truth is lies and lies are truth. Democracy is dictatorship, food is starvation, medicine poison, and justice injustice. Child protection is child trafficking, and to serve and protect is to extort and destroy.

Also, when it comes to climate-change deceptions, hot is cold and cold is hot. If you find this last element jolting, note how the climate-change narrative has followed the same playbook as COVID: take a threat that is negligible or non-existent and inflate it into a harbinger of planetary doom. To bring about such overthrows of reason requires a constant barrage of indoctrination, censorship, propaganda, fear-mongering, and psychological torture, areas where so-called 'intelligence agencies' have long honed their dark arts.

With such intense attack in the arena of ideas, and with ideas being broadcast through the invisible medium of the air, might you infer this is a spiritual battle too? Do you sense a malevolent spiritual entity or network behind the scenes? Might you call that entity Satan or Lucifer? And if such an impostor set up a throne and called himself God or Messiah, would that not be the king of all inversions?

Still, I venture that you and I are so *over* state-sanctioned lies by now that the tyrants have given up trying to persuade us. Yet they must still convince *themselves*, if only to quell any protest from Conscience. "Uncertain way of gain," to quote Shakespeare's *Richard III*, "but I am in/ So far in blood that sin will pluck on sin./ Tear-falling pity dwells not in this eye" (IV.ii).

Meanwhile, if you harbour distrust of Christians, bear in mind that not all who *call* themselves Christians are truly members of the Body of Christ. Some are wolves in sheep's clothing or, calling on Shakespeare again, beautiful tyrants, fiends angelical, dove-feathered ravens, honorable villains, serpent hearts (*Romeo and Juliet*, III.ii). And some are false prophets, eager to share what "God told me."

Beware, too, of 'Controlled Opposition', those tasked with drawing dissidents into a 'Limited Hangout' that refuses to look at deeper and more horrid realities. Keep your wits about you, practise discernment, and sniff out the spiritual rot of these whitewashed tombs full of dead men's bones (*Matthew* 23:27).

But seek out those who genuinely *are* in Christ and who have chosen his ultimate authority over the false authority of men. We Christians may be all that is standing between you and annihilation. Have you noticed how Christian voices have taken the lead in recent years in denouncing and exposing the perpetrators? When, since the days of Moses or Joshua, has there been such a need for a fierce Christian army?

Do not resent your protectors, who are already paying a price for our faith. As Harrison Smith observed in a May 2024 interview with Maria Zeee, Christianity is under attack today because it impedes the totalitarian agenda...

> "It makes it hard to control people. It makes it hard to deceive and manipulate. When the whole society is sincerely righteous and desires truth and desires justice, then you can't get away with things very easily. You have to have a whole system that's corrupt and fallen, and then it makes it easy to scam, it makes it easy to get one over. They want the dog-eat-dog world where they can screw somebody over and destroy them and suffer no consequences. So Christianity is a barrier to control, it's a barrier to oppression. **It gives you something higher than earthly authority, and that naturally pisses off the earthly authority**" (emphasis mine).

Speaking of earthly authority, I will not pin my hopes on a political solution to our woes. The *Declaration of Independence* doesn't tell us to "abolish" this or that political party or political candidate, nor does it call on us to favour one traitor, despot, pussy-grabber, or paedophile over another. No, it is our "duty" to abolish any *form* of Government that is destructive of Life, Liberty, and the Pursuit of Happiness.

Many more people are aware now that political parties oppose each other in only the most superficial ways, but when it comes to matters that really affect our lives, they are firm allies in trying to despoil us. As Mike Adams observed, in an April 2024 article,...

> "The Democrats have actively destroyed this once-great nation, but the Republicans were either wholly complicit or stood by and did nothing while the arsonists set fire to the pillars of our constitutional republic. As is now obvious to anyone paying attention, we no longer have a functioning civil society in the United States of America. We have a failed government, failed election integrity, a failed justice system, a failed counterfeit currency, fake corporate media, fake war propaganda, a failed educational system, and a weaponized system of science and medicine that literally develops and deploys biological weapons against the American people."

Why do politicians act in concert against us, no matter what party they're in? Because, deep down, they're not really Democrats or Republicans, Conservatives or Labour, or whatever. These are just convenient labels for their sham political theatre. No, they serve but one party, and that is the party of Freemasonry. According to Bible scholar David Carrico, in a November 2019 episode of *Now You See TV*,...

> "If you look at the Democratic Party and the Republican Party, if you look close enough, both are Masonically controlled... These two American political parties, they are just the expression of two Masonic philosophies that both have the same ultimate goal, and that will be the New World Order."

That's why petitions and protests are useless when you're dealing with them. So too are polls when they have no compunction about rigging elections. As Max Igan observes, "There's nobody you can vote in. There's nobody you can vote out. There's no political remedy to this system."

True, Max. There is no political remedy, but other remedies are at hand. That's why I have written this book, a battle manual for warriors determined to overthrow tyrants of every stripe. One way or another, we must reclaim our Sovereignty, our freedom of action, even our freedom of thought. I do not mean a 'Great Reset' such as our enemies have conceived, but at least a Great Reckoning to restore Justice and consequence for the innumerable Crimes Against Humanity unleashed against Mankind. When, like a mighty river Justice returns, the overlords will be destroyed as surely as Pharaoh and his chariots were destroyed when they chased Moses into the Red Sea (*Exodus* 14:26-28). I trust this book shall serve as armour and weapon in the battle ahead, for battle it is, and battle it will be.

Abdiel LeRoy

INTRODUCTION TO 'KNOW YOUR FINANCIAL RIGHTS'

BOOK 3 IN 'BATTLE MANUALS FOR FREEDOM'

And each in the cell of himself is almost convinced of his freedom.

— W.H. AUDEN, *IN MEMORY OF W.B. YEATS*

WE HAVE BEEN HORRIBLY RIPPED OFF!

In your heart, you know this. From dawn to dusk, from cradle to grave, we have been tax-farmed, fined, and fleeced. We have been stripped of our dignity, prodded, probed, and poked, and ordered about by half-wits who have not one shred of courage, integrity, or truth in their hearts. Brothers and Sisters, I have had enough, and this *Battle Manual for Freedom* is my response.

I wrote *Know Your Medical Rights* (originally titled *The COVID Protocols: Upholding Your Rights in Authoritarian Times*) as a weapon against the medical tyranny that, starting in 2020, sought to desecrate our constitutional protections. Job done, or so I thought.

But as we now know, COVID was just the opening assault. We are also being assailed by poisons in our food, water, earth, and air; engineered shortages, and sabotage; radiation and energy weapons; along with war, assassination programs, fabricated emergencies, and false-flag terrorism.

Among other forms of attack are: lawless legislation and destructive regulation; impositions of a counterfeit righteousness; censorship, propaganda, fear-mongering, and indoctrination; monitoring and surveillance; digital imprisonment and technocracy; demoralization and destruction of hope; separation, isolation, and division; demolition of the family, culture, and meritocracy; stolen elections; weaponized immigration; ecological devastation and pollution (nothing to do with carbon-dioxide, by the way); and overall treason by politicians, bureaucrats, agencies, corporations, courts, and police.

To counter all this, I wrote the next book, *Know Your Lawful Rights*, but even then, the work was not finished, for the predator class are coming at us with all manner of financial attack too, including murderous levels of taxation, inflation, debt, and confiscation of assets and property. Meanwhile, bank runs, bank failures, and bank freezes are looming, and even bank bail-ins, where they just help themselves to the contents of your account.

On the other side of this obliteration, our enemies plan central-bank digital currencies (CBDC), where they can reward your behaviour if they like it, and penalize your behaviour and speech if they don't, and make further deductions on a whim without giving you recourse. Hence this third and final book in the series, *Know Your Financial Rights*.

I recall the horrifying scenes of pallets of cash left behind when the U.S. military bolted from Afghanistan in 2021. However worthless, that paper represents the toil of millions of Americans whose life's work has been squandered by a vampiric cabal hell-bent on enriching themselves while destroying us.

We know in our hearts we were not put on this Earth to supply these parasites. We who are in Christ also remember that his yoke is easy and his burden is light (*Matthew* 11:28-30). Like the kin of Moses longing to break free from Egypt and its state-sanctioned death cult, we too long for our Exodus and restoration of our Birthright. May this book sever the chains that held us, especially the spiritual ones, for if our minds are free, our reality shall follow. This requires us to dispel the delusions and mind-tricks that have been played on us for centuries, even millennia.

When it comes to solutions, I do not claim to be the tip of the spear; others have done more battle than I. Rather, my contribution is to bring into coherence the myriad fragments of wisdom, analysis, and experience that are out there, and above all to clarify them. As I said, Christ's burden is light, and that includes the financial one. If solutions are too complicated for the layman to grasp, I will simplify them if possible and discard them if not.

Nor am I am setting out to prescribe one-size-fits-all remedies. "There is no magic bullet," to quote Si 'the Spaniard' of youandyourcash.com, when I attended one of his seminars in England. "You're the magic bullet." You will pick and choose from the tools at your disposal and play to your particular strengths.

That is our key advantage as we undermine, obstruct, and overthrow the evil plans of financial despots. Wise as serpents, we are inventing strategies and approaches so numerous and varied that the enemy cannot possibly find an answer to all of them. Compared to the one-government, one-narrative, one-opinion, one-way, one-rule, one-religion, one-food, one-health, one-medicine, and one-currency brigade opposing us, we are a motley crew, but I celebrate that. As C.S. Lewis wrote, "Good, as it ripens, becomes continually more different, not only from evil, but from other good."1

Now, as you may be aware, I just quoted Scripture with "wise as serpents" (*Matthew* 10:16). Some readers have complained that I speak too much of spiritual battle in this book series and about the victory of Christ and his prophets over Satan's schemes and schemers.

To which I say, deal with it. If you think you're going to get through the battles ahead against foes who are themselves deeply religious and who are supernaturally allied with infernal forces, then you will be easy meat for their murderous agenda. Also, if my offering is good fruit from a holy root, it were blasphemous to reject the tree that produced it.

Jesus—or Yeshua or Yehusha if you prefer—gave us

authority to overcome all the power of the enemy (*Luke* 10:19). In addition to this spiritual authority, we have the authority of logic because, as the documentary *Strawman* reminds us, "Government is a creation of man, and a creation of man can never be above man."

This authority equates to that of the Lawful realm, meaning that which the Most High bestows, over the Legal realm, which is what men write, revise, and repeal. Which raises the question: Why bother operating in the Legal arena at all—with its politicians, bureaucrats, autocrats, and technocrats, its corporations and courts, so-called lawyers and police? Only because they have a nasty habit of showing up where they're not wanted and not needed. We are to put them back in their inferior places and disabuse them of their power-hungry ambitions to play God in the lives of others.

As Shakespeare observed, "All the world's a stage/ And all the men and women merely players" (*As You Like It*, II.vii.). Sometimes, we are called to put on a costume and play a role in the Theatre of the Legal, but we are not *of* the Legal. When the play is over, we take off the costume, resume our higher life, and leave behind those who are trapped in the Legal illusion and think it is real and all that there is.

Much love,
Abdiel LeRoy

BATTLE MANUALS FOR FREEDOM

GENI.US/RIGHTS

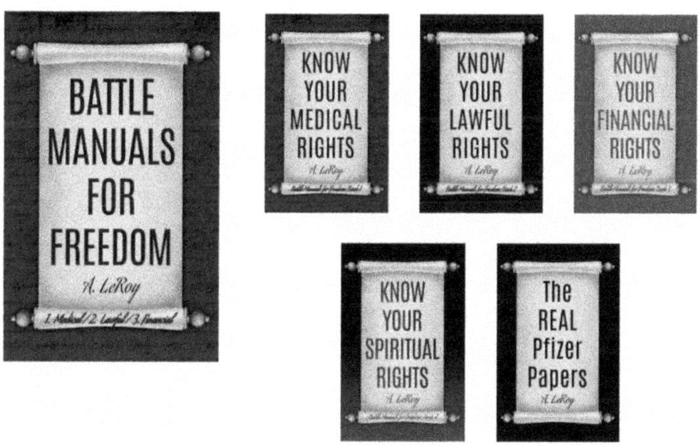

Book 1: *Know Your Medical Rights*

Book 2: *Know Your Lawful Rights*

Book 3: *Know Your Financial Rights*

Book 4: *Know Your Spiritual Rights*

FROM THE AUTHOR

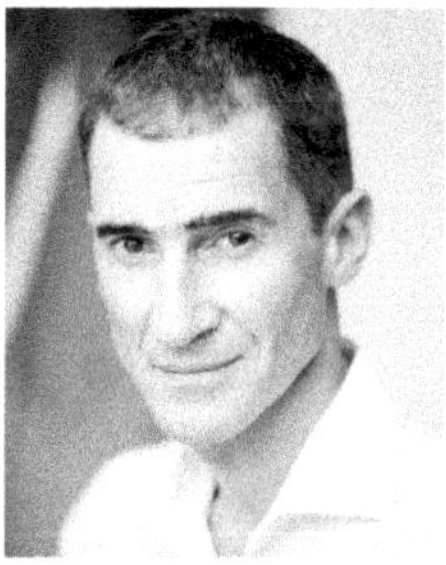

Thank you for reading my book, and if you have found value in it, I'd welcome your review wherever you usually buy books. A couple of sentences would suffice.

Also, if I've missed something important, or a link doesn't work, or you find some other glitch, let me know. I am quick to make adjustments when readers point them out to me. My email is RenewedTestament@protonmail.com.

Meanwhile, if you'd like to keep up to date with my goings-on, you can find a mailing-list sign-up on the Home page of my website, PoetProphet.com. I also post occasional videos on 'alternative' video-hosting sites such as Bastyon, BitChute, and Brighteon, and I frequently put articles on Substack at *The Poet's Eye* (though I have been 'demonetized' there.)

I don't bother with TikTok any more after it savaged my content with censorship, strikes, and shadow-banning, and I gave up on Facebook, YouTube, and Twitter long ago.

If you would like to support my work, the best way is

to buy my books and leave reviews. My other published titles, listed below, encompass novelas, non-fiction, memoir, poetry, and epic poetry.

Abdiel LeRoy
December 2024

EXTRAS

THE 'MEDICAL-FREEDOM MOVEMENT' COULD GET US ALL KILLED!

To you leaders of the so-called 'Medical-Freedom Movement'. Whose side are you on, really? Your lazy thinking and wilful ignorance have cost untold numbers of lives. You repeat the same old strategies and tired old phrases that merely trim the weeds of medical tyranny while allowing its poisonous root to spread. Your errors could get us all killed.

Your most dangerous mistake is to base opposition to forced medicine not on the solid ground that it is eternally unlawful, but on the shifting sands of data and statistics. You say something to the effect of, "This disease, or that variant, is too mild to warrant this or that measure." Or, "You shouldn't have a mandate when there is possible risk."

You utter, utter fools! What you are saying is that you'd be absolutely fine with forced medicine if the circumstances were different, such as a more serious disease, or if a safer countermeasure were produced.

Your stupidity is breathtaking. If Rights are expendable depending on conditions on the ground, or depending on statistics that so-called experts tell you, then they're not rights at all; they're flimsy conveniences.

So fuck the 'Science', and uphold our Rights! Forced medicine is eternally unlawful yesterday, today, and forever. And no emergency, whether real or perceived or invented, removes one single medical Right or any other type of Right.

Even if there were a plague on the scale of the Black Death that wiped out half the population, and even if there were some medical intervention proven to be 100% safe and 100% effective, no-one ever, under any circumstances, would have authority to impose it.

And here's your second biggest mistake: that you never defend medical confidentiality. The ***Hippocratic Oath*** doesn't just say, "First, do no harm" and, "I will administer no deadly medicine," it also says, "I will not divulge." And that principle of Confidentiality is enshrined in international Rights declarations and the **Fourth Amendment** to ***The Constitution of the United States of America***.

Yet you're absolutely fine with the government, or an employer, or a travel company knowing your medical status or your vaccination status. It's none of their goddamn business. No-one has to divulge their medical status, and if you're not divulging your medical status, no-one can discriminate against you or persecute you on the basis of it.

Also, if they don't know your medical status, there's no need to apply for a so-called exemption. The word "No" is exemption enough. It always has been, and always will be, exemption enough.

I'm telling you to be a **CONSTITUTIONAL EXTREMIST**. Anything less, and you're dead!

Here's your third mistake. You are forgetting to tell people that, as enshrined in the ***Universal Declaration on Bioethics and Human Rights***, along with many more medical codes, we have the Right to **refuse diagnostic measures**, including tests, not just purportedly preventive measures such as masks, injections, quarantines, and lockdowns.

If you had told people that before they went into the charnel houses that hospitals have become, how many more could have been saved? Armed with this information, patients would refuse the supposed 'COVID' tests that have been channeling them into corridors of death and the hospital protocols designed to kill.

But you didn't tell them that, did you? And you're still not telling them. How many lives have been lost through your complicit silence?

Fourth mistake: Lawyers staying inside your little legislative boxes, whinging that you can't go after Big Pharma or doctors or politicians or bureaucrats because they have 'legal immunity'. Do you not realize that all the Acts and statutes that confer this supposed 'legal immunity' are nothing more than corporate contracts that only one party has agreed to and only one party has signed?!

You and I, we the People, were never consulted about these contracts, did not write these contracts, did not negotiate these contracts, didn't even read these contracts, and we certainly didn't sign these contracts. Without our signature, these corporate contracts are not worth the air they're written on. Yet you lawyers are taking them as gospel.

And why, lawyers, instead of drawing on universal and international constitutions, declarations, and conventions, are you confining yourselves within the walls of a shrinking domestic legislative box that provides cover for atrocity and injustice, while you echo the oppressors by mislabeling their tyrannical codes 'law'?

Fifth mistake. Expecting any salvation from a political party or a political candidate, such as Florida governor, Ron DeSantis, just because he throws you a few bones, while you overlook the state statutes he has signed that glaringly promote medical tyranny, including forced quarantine and forced vaccination (SB 2006 and SB 7014), or that desecrate the **First Amendment** (HB 269 and HB 741)?

Remember the duty conferred on us by the ***Declaration of Independence***. It doesn't tell us to abolish a political party or a political candidate. It tells us to abolish any *form* of Government that is destructive of Life, Liberty, and the Pursuit of Happiness. And that includes a form of Government that offers a political duopoly where both sides are united in trying to destroy us.

Sixth mistake. You lean disproportionately on the Nuremberg Code, which applies to experimental medicine, while overlooking other international Rights protections and medical codes that apply to all medicine, whether experimental or not. They include the ***Universal Declaration on Bioethics and Human Rights***, the ***Siracusa Principles***, the **NHS *Code of Practice***, and the **NHS *Constitution***. Where are you going to go when the authorities, the powers-that-shouldn't-be, say, "It's no longer experimental because we've fully approved it. So Nuremberg doesn't apply any more." Where are you going to go?

Finally, you're using the enemy's definitions of words, such as what 'pandemic' means or what 'vaccine' means.

Here's an example that includes the most egregious mistakes. In January 2023, Children's Health Defense (CHD) rejoiced that the New York State Supreme Court ruled against the state's vaccine mandate for healthcare workers. So far, so good, but...

The judge didn't overturn the mandate because it was inherently unlawful, which it is; he did it because it came from an executive order and was not voted on by the legislature. Meaning what? That if the governor can't be sole tyrant, the legislature can? Does an unlawful mandate become valid if only it follows the prescribed procedure?

The court also decided that the mandate was "arbitrary and capricious" on the basis that the "vaccines" do not stop transmission of the "virus"! Meaning what? That if another medical product is conjured that they say *does* stop transmission, you'd be fine with forcing it on people?

CHD's lawyer said that if the mandate "can't stop the spread of COVID, then it's just arbitrary and irrational." Meaning what? That if a product *could* stop the spread of a disease, then forcing it suddenly *would* become rational? Is this what they taught you in law school?

Oh, and she talked about the mandate causing a staffing shortage in New York hospitals. Why are you making all these peripheral arguments that don't address the core tyranny? You are leaving the door open for future tyranny!

Afterwards, CHD president Mary Holland said, "We are thrilled by this critical win against a COVID vaccine mandate, correctly finding that any such mandate at this stage, given current knowledge, is arbitrary."

"At this stage?" "Given current knowledge"? What is she thinking? No! The mandate is arbitrary, period, end of story, eternally, in every circumstance, at every stage, and whatever the current levels of knowledge or ignorance!

Holland's statement echoes another hollow slogan we've heard in 'medical-freedom' circles. "Where there is risk, there must be choice." Again, you're conferring on medical tyrants a false authority to remove choice when they claim there is no risk.

The Children's Health Defense lawyer also complained that the mandate didn't have a religious exemption. So you'd be fine with forcing it on people who don't claim to follow a religion?

My friends. This is a hollow, hollow victory, because you didn't address the core desecrations at work. Again, I say, be a **CONSTITUTIONAL EXTREMIST**. You cannot mandate medicine of any kind, at any time, or in any circumstances.

So before you get more people killed, understand and uphold…

1. All medical coercion is outlawed eternally, whatever the circumstances.
2. Medical confidentiality is eternally sacred.
3. The word "No" is exemption enough.
4. Refuse the tests!
5. Bring Justice, regardless of Acts and statutes, and stop bending the knee to unlawful legislation.

Without all these, all you're doing is nibbling around the edges of medical tyranny but never striking at the root. And that, as I've said, could get us all killed!

Abdiel LeRoy

THE AWAKENING

Many were the souls that swept past me, their screams a vast orchestra of terror. They were flying, most of them, but there was no joy in their flight, only anguish and dread. I realized I too was mid-air, my soul also consumed with terror. And then…

That I was dead. We were all dead. Some terrible event had occurred to set us all adrift at once, dislocated spirits, suddenly removed from all we knew and loved, even our reassuring contact with the earth.

Yet, even in this state of limbo, untethered to hope, love, or connection, I began to sense that all was not lost, that we were not forever doomed to languish in agony of soul.

Some screamed still, but others, as I, began to settle and become quiet. We were waiting, and as the lamentations abated, they were replaced by a sound like rushing waters, accompanied by something like a warm breeze that brought comfort, as a golden glow began to permeate the gloom.

By now, all voices had ceased, and each of us became still, floating in air.

Then the glow brightened until it became almost too bright to behold. A flash of gold, and I found myself facing a great wingèd being so dazzling that I felt I would be consumed in his fire.

But when our eyes met, he immediately slipped into another state, his wings folded, and he became an outline in the whiteness, a moving sketch in ink, who seemed to sit before me. By now, all awareness of others was gone, and he and I sat face-to-face, as in private meeting.

But when he opened his mouth to speak, such a deafening roar came forth that once again I was put to terror. I motioned to scream myself, but no sound came forth.

Then the apparition, seeming almost as alarmed at the sound of his own voice as I, immediately put his hand to his mouth.

"Sorry about that," he said. "I'm new at this." His voice was gentle, deep, and reassuring.

Yet I was still too shocked to reply.

"Allow me to introduce myself," he continued. "I am Uriel. I stand in the presence of God."

At this, I took a deep breath as relief flooded my soul, and it was the first time since... since what shall I call it? My transmutation? My passage into another state of being?... that I even became aware that I had breath to breathe.

"I... I... I..."

"Yes, what you've experienced does tend to render mortals speechless at first, but I dare say you'll get the hang of it."

"You're Uriel?"

"Yes."

"I've heard of you. Aren't you Regent of the Sun? But you said you're new at this. So this is the first time you've..."

" 'Conveyed', we call it."

" 'Conveyed'? What does that mean?"

"Well, the battlefront's been a bit quiet of late. Not that the war in Heaven is any less intense, mind you. It's just that there's a lot more subtle stuff going on at the moment—intelligence-gathering, espionage, that sort of thing—so I thought I'd give conveyance a go. I've gone through all the training and made sure to fold my wings away when I approached you, become more human-like, and veil the fireglow. It's just my voice I forgot to change, and gave us *both* a fright. Again, please excuse."

"Um, I still don't know what 'conveyance' is."

"Ah yes, well, conveyance is when we come to souls newly released from their bodies..."

" 'Newly released from their bodies?' So I *am* dead."

"Hmm," said the angel, tilting his hand from side to side in a gesture of equivocation. "Your condition remains to be resolved, but in any case, you have nothing to fear."

"I see."

"No you don't, not really, but you will."

"So what happens now?"

"First, I need to introduce you to someone."

With that, I heard beautiful birdsong, followed by the sudden appearance of a little robin, russet of breast, tawny of tail and wings, who flew to some vaguely discernible perch between me and the angel.

Oh if I could describe his melody—so rich, so complex, so virtuous, but most of all, calming and reassuring. I had seen this little fellow often in my countryside walks in England and in its hedgerows and gardens, his presence always welcoming, always gladdening my heart. I had ever delighted in his song, but now I could discern its meaning, which I will try to set down here, however imperfectly.

"*I am thy messenger, and always was,*
Watched over you from Heaven and on Earth,
Prepared the way for you, from first to last,
And I was there to celebrate your birth."

Taking my lead from his manner of speech, I asked, "What is thy name?"

"You know my name," the bird replied, "for it is yours, honored and celebrated in your epic verse."

I gasped.

"I dared to hope it would be you
Who heard the prophet in a former age,
An age of wickedness, as is this one,
With new atrocity on History's page."

"Of such atrocity I come to speak,
An intercessor now divinely sent
To counter Mankind's fear and greed and hate.
All creatures of the Earth I represent.

"Soon shall my kind from tree branch disappear,
No longer shall our song herald God's call.
Birds, bees, and butterflies, from briar to brook,
Man will not stop 'til he has slaughtered all."

I knew his message to be true, the forces of destruction to be relentless and implacable, even slowing them down a superhuman challenge, let alone stopping them or repairing the devastation left in their rapacious wake.

"Heavy my heart to hear these dismal tidings,
That man's defilement of land, air, and sea,
Shall so persist as to extinguish hope,
Its dimming flame snuffed out eternally."

"But, man of God, this is not writ in stone.
If you and others like you overcome
The earthly powers now wielding their destruction,
The Will of God on Earth may yet be done."

"But it appears that I have left this Earth,"
I countered, "that my soul from body's split.
How then may I bring Heaven's Will to Earth
Without the vehicle to channel it?"

Now the robin turned to Uriel, who all this while had listened in silence to our conversation. The angel interjected:

"It's up to you now. I am come to give you three choices. In an instant, I could summon a chariot of fire to take you Heaven-ward and to the eternal realms. Or, with your namesake, you could fly the skies above the Earth and gladden receptive hearts. Or, your third choice, to return to Earth as your mortal self and enact the mission just described. In any case, you will be beloved and blessed of the Eternal Father, and your choice today can neither increase nor diminish that."

Uriel now nodded to the robin who, taking his cue, flew out of our circle, piping new melodies as he left. And once more, I was alone with the angel, to whom I thought aloud:

"Better it is to be with the Lord, to follow in Elijah's wake to Heaven immediately, or to take wing with the robin, but in either case, I'd leave behind such a scene of devastation. I love this Earth and all its beauty. And though a better place awaits, I cannot abandon it now. I must go back."

"Then be it so!" said the angel.

He immediately transformed, his eyes blazing like fire, a flash of gold again, then vanished in an instant. I found myself lying on a windswept heath, staring up at a pale sky. I touched my chest to verify that I was man and flesh again, a beating heart within. Shakily, I got to my feet, and saw that others were beginning to stir around me.

They were obviously bewildered, yet I detected in

their demeanour quiet resolve. I knew instinctively that they had just experienced a revelation similar to mine. In silence, we walked toward each other until we were a small group.

"For Heaven and Earth?" I asked.

"For Heaven and Earth," all replied.

And it was so.

Abdiel LeRoy

ONE DOCUMENT AND TWO OFFICIAL STATEMENTS TELL YOU ALL YOU NEED TO KNOW

Overwhelmed with information? Swamped with videos, links, books, and articles that underline the reality of medical genocide? Don't know how to convey the horrid truths to friends and family who have short attention spans and conditioned beliefs? Here's my suggestion...

One document—and two official statements—say it all...

The document was available to regulators in May 2021 and to the public in November 2021. I call it, *The Cumulative Analysis Report,* to avoid reeling off its full unwieldy title (*5.3.6 CUMULATIVE ANALYSIS OF POST-AUTHORIZATION ADVERSE EVENT REPORTS OF PF-07302048 (BNT162B2) RECEIVED THROUGH 28-FEB-2021)*. You can find it at https://phmpt.org/wp-content/uploads/2022/04/reissue_5.3.6-postmarketing-experience.pdf

You may have heard of it. It’s famous, or rather infamous. It collates adverse-event reports that Pfizer received, unsolicited—and therefore vastly under-reported—between public rollout of 'vaccines' in December 2020 until the end of February 2021. It's a relatively short document and not hard to comprehend.

Among the key facts...

1. Of 28 potential babies of injected mothers, 26 DIED BY SPONTANEOUS ABORTION, and one by neonatal death. There was only one "normal outcome."

2. Small children were being injected way under the age of authorization at the time, especially in the U.K.

3. The document counted 1,223 post-injection deaths among all age groups.

4. The Appendix lists 1,294 'adverse events of special interest'. These are categories of potential harm that Pfizer knew about in advance.

Now for the two official statements…

GOV.UK

Home > COVID-19 > Health and wellbeing during COVID-19

Press release

Unvaccinated mothers urge pregnant women to get jabbed

Powerful new video shows their experiences of severe COVID-19 during pregnancy.

From: Department of Health and Social Care
Published 4 December 2021

The first is a Dec. 4, 2021 press release from the U.K. National 'Health' Service urging pregnant women to get jabbed. Among nine uses of the word 'safe' to describe the injections, it quotes then Vaccines Minister Maggie Throup saying, "The COVID-19 vaccines are safe and effective for pregnant women and I urge everyone to get their vaccines as soon as they can to secure this significant protection."

Vaccines Minister Maggie Throup said:

" Nearly 1 in 5 COVID-19 patients who are most critically ill are pregnant women who have not been vaccinated, which shows just how important it is that expectant mothers get the vaccine to keep themselves and their babies safe.

" Over 81,000 pregnant women have so far received their first dose, with 65,000 being double-jabbed, which is fantastic, but there's still more to be done.

" The COVID-19 vaccines are safe and effective for pregnant women and I urge everyone to get their vaccines as soon as they can to secure this significant protection."

These statements by Throup and others came AFTER

public release of the Pfizer document showing the carnage happening to babies.

The second official statement comes from that oily operative, Dr. Peter Marks, head of the Center for Biologics Evaluation and Research (CBER) at the FDA. On May 19, 2022, now MORE THAN A YEAR after the FDA received the Pfizer document showing devastation to babies, he publicly stated in a YouTube video,...

"Pregnant or breastfeeding women can certainly receive a COVID-19 vaccine... There is currently no evidence that any vaccines, including COVID-19 vaccines, cause fertility problems in either women or men."

I hope these observations help. I have written several books on COVID atrocities, along with poems and articles, but I keep coming back to the same document and to these two statements as they encapsulate the atrocities without requiring too much investigation by the information overloaded.

Abdiel LeRoy

A COVID AMNESTY IS EVIL AND UNGODLY

The COVID tyrants, and their media servants, seem to be pinning their hopes on the idea that Christians forgive, no matter what. They seem to think we will pardon their crimes with neither repercussion nor reproach and leave them at large to go about their next round of Satanic business.

It doesn't work like that. It never did. And we have a blueprint of exemplary forgiveness from Joseph in the Old Testament. It goes like this (excerpted from my book series, *The Gourmet Gospel*)...

Joseph's brothers threatened his life and sold him into slavery at the age of 17 (*Genesis* 37:18-28). More than 20 years later, when he is Pharaoh's right-hand man in Egypt, those brothers appear before him on the verge of destitution (*Genesis* 42). He recognizes them, but they do not know who he is.

What example does Joseph give us here? Does he

immediately declare himself to them, embrace them, and throw open the granaries of Egypt to his former tormentors? No. He continues to conceal his identity while putting them through a series of tests to see if their hearts have changed.

The first evidence of this is when he overhears them saying, "Surely we are being punished because of our brother. We saw how distressed he was when he pleaded with us for his life, but we would not listen. That's why this distress has come upon us." This moves Joseph to tears, though he weeps them in secret.

Forgiveness has begun, but it is not yet complete. More tests follow, as Joseph sends his brothers back to Canaan to fetch the youngest, Benjamin, while keeping another, Simeon, hostage. When they return, and Joseph sees Benjamin, his only full brother among the group (the rest being half-brothers), he again weeps in secret.

Final proof of his brothers' repentance, however, comes after Joseph has Benjamin framed for the theft of a silver cup, as the group set out for Canaan a second time. The penalty for Benjamin is to become an Egyptian slave. At this point, the ten other brothers could simply have abandoned the youngest to bondage in Egypt, as they had done with Joseph all those years ago, but instead go back to face the music together.

Finally, when Judah offers to pay the penalty of slavery himself by taking Benjamin's place, Joseph is overcome and can no longer conceal his identity. He sees the repentance of his brothers, their readiness to take upon themselves the suffering they had once inflicted, and declares himself to them. Now bursts his mighty heart; forgiveness is complete.

In this example, forgiveness goes hand in hand with the repentance of the offender; the wronged and the wronger cooperate. The crime is not overlooked, whitewashed, or generalized, not diminished, downplayed, or diluted. Joseph says to his brothers, "I am your brother, Joseph, the one you sold into Egypt… You intended to harm me, but God intended it for good."

Joseph's story also demonstrates that forgiveness is not just a religious concept but a human capacity, built into our nature, and once bestowed inwardly, can find its outer expression. Had Joseph been too hasty in his forgiveness, he would not only have robbed his own heart of its time and process, but denied his brothers the gift of repentance.

Yet most Christians put the cart of outward forgiveness before the horse of inward forgiveness. And how many would dare do so "unchristian" a thing as frame his own brother for a theft? What emerges from Joseph's story is a skilfully choreographed dance of forgiveness, a poetic drama written by the Holy Spirit in human hearts.

So too, in Shakespeare's *The Tempest*. At the start of the play, Prospero relates to his daughter Miranda that he had been Duke of Milan until his own brother, Antonio, usurped the kingdom, betrayed it to the king of Naples, and set the two of them adrift in a condemned vessel to die.

But they survived, and Prospero, using his magical

powers, assisted by the spirit Ariel, imprisons his would-be murderers and confronts them with their crimes. Only when he is satisfied they are "full of sorrow and dismay" does he conclude, "The rarer action is/ In virtue than in vengeance. They being penitent,/ ... Go release them, Ariel" (V.i.27-30).

In both cases, the two maltreated men bring their tormentors within their own power and discover the repentant condition of their hearts before forgiveness is bestowed.

Therefore, when the unrepentant tormentors of our race come to us today demanding we wipe from remembrance their crimes against humanity so they may have a blank cheque to commit fresh atrocity, they only multiply their culpability. Rather, let us heed the commands given us in *Revelation* concerning Babylon, giving back to them as they have given, paying back double for what they have done, and giving them as much torture and grief as they doled out to our kin (18:4-7). Amnesty be damned!

Abdiel LeRoy, November 2023

KLAUS AND THE DEVIL

The old man wore his favourite garment for this much anticipated meeting, a long black robe with billowing sleeves and thick lapels that reflected the dim candlelight of the temple. Much blood had been spilled through the night onto the checkered tiles beneath his feet, for the cult devotees had done their job well. Since dusk, they had butchered long and hard with their sacrificial knives, while others watched, chanting and swaying in unison. And once the last drop of blood had been extracted, they practised upon each other astonishing feats of defilement.

These scenes were still playing in the mind of the man as he made his way across the alternating black and white tiles, but the temple was still again now. The floor had been hastily mopped, though the fetid odour of body fluids hung in the air. The altar itself had not been touched, and still steamed with the offal of sacrifice, dripping steadily onto the tiles beneath.

Would his shoes be stained? the man wondered. They were extremely rare and expensive, and he considered removing them before moving closer, but then he reasoned that, as they were a deep red colour to begin with, blood spatters wouldn't make much difference.

Behind the altar hung two braided curtains, fringed with gold, a slight gap between them, and a red glow pulsing from behind. The man trembled with anticipation.

"Klaus," said a drawling voice.

"Master," the man whispered back in fearful awe.

"Your work tonight was…"

"Master?"

"Satisfactory."

"Zank you, Master," said the man, though he had hoped for higher praise than this. "To bring you pleasure is our delight."

"And you did. And you did. Danke, Klaus," replied the voice.

"Bitte, Meister." He loved it when his lord addressed him in his native tongue.

"But now, we have other matters to discuss, do we not, Klaus?"

"As you wish, Master."

"Oh, be assured, I do wish. I wish very much."

"Yes, Master."

"So how's everything going with the Project, Klaus?"

"We are making good progress."

"Are you, Klaus? Are you really?"

There was something in the tone of this question that

unnerved the man. A chill passed down his body as he replied, "Yes, Master. Many have died."

"Hmm. What's your definition of 'many', Klaus?"

"Tens of millions."

"Oh dear, Klaus. 'Tens of millions,' you say. I'm afraid that won't do. There are still billions of humans running around the planet, yet you call that 'good progress.' I mean, yes you've managed to kill off some millions with the Weapon, and others have perished from famine, war, poison, and so on, but you're still woefully short of the target. Did I not instruct you to get the world's population down to 500 million? Did you not see the Georgia Guidestones before they were blown up?"

"Of course I am aware of zem, Master."

"Then you will also be aware that you are still several billion bodies short of the extermination target."

"We will do better, Master."

"Hmm."

"And ze Weapon hasn't reached its full effect yet."

"Ah yes, that brings me to another matter, Klaus, old boy. About the timing of that effect. Why did you kill off so many so quickly?"

"Master, was not extermination ze goal?"

"Yes, Klaus, extermination was *ze* goal."

Hearing this hint of mockery from his lord unnerved the man even more. For a moment, his cheek spasmed uncontrollably, until he managed to overcome his nerves.

"A for effort, Klaus," the voice continued, "but why did you kill and injure with such immediate effect? You see, with all these people keeling over just after the shot, and many of those caught on camera, you've alerted people to the danger."

"Zis was an oversight, my lord, but only because some of my colleagues were overzealous in zeir duty."

"Ha! Overzealous, you call it? Downright reckless, I'd say. You were supposed to install gradual decay into their bodies so that we might have plausible deniability, but now, with all these videos circulating of athletes and news anchors dropping like flies, people falling under trains and what have you, you have badly tipped our hand. What an appalling lack of discipline..."

"Master, I will put it right..."

"I haven't finished. Not only did you alert people to the danger prematurely, you robbed us of our pleasure in the slow torture of our Enemy's beloved creatures."

"Forgive me, Master."

"Forgive you? What do you take me for, Klaus, to suppose forgiveness is in *my* nature?"

The man had no answer, and his cheek spasmed again, and this time it took him longer to bring it back under control.

"And another question," the voice went on. "Why did you roll out the Weapon at the beginning of 2021? You made it stupidly easy for them to chart excess deaths on a year-by-year basis. Why didn't you introduce it mid-way through the year so that you could fudge the numbers better?

"We will do better with ze next pandemic."

"*Ze* next pandemic, eh? Perhaps, perhaps."

"Yes, we have ze next variant ready to go."

"Oh Klaus, now you're starting to bore me. That narrative has been going rapidly downhill since, what was it, Omicron? And then what came after, Ninja or some such? And then you got really sexy with, what, BA1 and BA2? Listen, Klaus, old fellow. How are people going to be fearful of some new variant if they can't even remember its name? Even I can't keep them all straight!"

"I understand, Master, but next we shall bring a new disease: Marburg, perhaps, or Ebola."

"They're hardly new, though, are they, Klaus?"

"But we have changed zem in ze laboratory."

"Ah! Have you now? More spike protein, perhaps? More snake venom? The problem is you have made people so distrustful after your premature kill spree that you've made it ever so much harder to mount another fear campaign. What is it those disgusting humans say? 'Fool me once...' and all of that? No, Klaus, on due reflection, I'm going to have to rethink my strategy. You and the World Economic Forum are really not fit for purpose."

A gasp of disbelief escaped from the old man's mouth, and even his best efforts could not keep his cheek spasms in check. "But, Master," he pleaded, "we did our best."

"Oh Klaus, you do amuse me. Did your best? You're starting to sound like a Christian. Our Enemy may be disposed to bestow his 'unmerited favour' on those who love him, in spite of their many failures, but surely you don't think *I'm* going to do that, do you? No, I'm going to get rid of the WEF and, for that matter, the United Nations and the World Health Organization. And I'm going to destroy them all by the hand of my real agent on Earth."

"But, my lord, am I not your agent?"

"Oh Klaus, don't be absurd. Your cover is blown, you're a laughing stock. No-one will believe you. No, the one I have appointed will appear as a saviour by going after the likes of you, but in the end will turn out to be an even worse tyrant than those he removes. Devilishly clever, don't you think, even if I do say so myself? Yes, we'll start with a soft kill at first, but it won't be long before he goes full Man-of-Lawlessness, if you get my drift. He will break you and your little Davos club, for so it is written. Nothing personal, you understand."

"But Master, all my years of service."

"Yes, I know. It's most unfortunate. All your years of service will, I fear, earn you more punishment at the hands of the Enemy. But do go on, Klaus. You're really quite entertaining."

"You promised me a reward!"

By now, the man had lost some of his fear as it gave way to deep-seated anger, resentment, and betrayal.

"Oh, that?" said the voice. "You mean you want me to extend your life? Not in my toolbox, old boy. Did you not drink enough adrenochrome then, Klaus?"

"Yes, but…"

"Did you not drink enough children? You and your chums got through quite a few tonight."

"Yes, but..."

"Ah, you mean… What was it you said in one of your boring little speeches? 'Fusion of our physical, digital, and biological identities.' Is that what you mean? You want your consciousness to be put in a chip and then keep yourself going in a machine or a skin or some such?"

"Not exactly, Master. You promised..."

"Stop right there, Klaussy Boy. I promised, did I? You do know what the Scriptures call me, don't you?"

"Yes, Master. You are called Lucifer."

"Well, yes, that's one name, but you seem to be forgetting something, Klaus, old boy."

"I don't follow, Master."

"Oh but I think you do, Klaus. Come on, you can do it. What else do they call me?"

"Ze Morning Star."

"Good. Keep going."

"Prince of ze Air, and ze Accuser."

"Bravo, Klaus, but you're still missing the key term here, old chap.

"You prowl like a lion."

"Yes, yes, yes, all of that, but you're still not hitting the mark there, Klaussy Boy, are you? Shall I spell it out for you? Shall I be plain? They call me Father of Lies, do they not?"

"Yes, Master."

"And do you suppose the Father of Lies makes promises and then keeps them? Who do you think I am? Our Enemy? Again, Klaus, you're sounding alarmingly like a Christian."

"Please, Master. Give me anozer chance. I shall bring more war, more deception, more famine, and we shall reach our target by 2030. We shall have more bioweapons, energy weapons, poison ze water, ze air, ze food, more radiation, more censorship, more surveillance, more legislation, cyber attacks, quarantine camps, more taxes and fines and fees to break ze will of ze people, und so on."

"Oh, Klaus, aren't you adorable? Bargaining with me to procure what? Mercy? I don't do mercy, Klaus. You should know that by now. 'The quality of mercy is not strained. It droppeth as the gentle rain from Heaven upon the place beneath.' Blah Blah Blah. Das ist Qwatsch, Klaus!"

The man's knees were shaking now, whether from fear or anger, an effect heightened by his interrogator's return to his native language, not to praise this time but in rebuke.

"Of course, I'm not into rain, either," the voice continued, "not normal rain, I mean. I go in more for tornadoes, hurricanes, earthquakes, floods, forest fires, you know the type of thing, what they foolishly call 'natural' disasters."

"Please, Master, I beg you..."

"Ah, that's more like it, Klaus, begging me, acknowledging my power over you, but it's still too late, old boy. You see, I've grown weary of you. Now run along and tell Justin to come in. He's waiting outside. I'm in need of some stimulation of a more physical nature, and he always proves most willing to oblige."

"Master, I could perform zis function if you wish."

"Oh, Klaus. The very thought. How revolting. Do I seem that desperate to you?"

"Zat's not what I mean. I mean I can do... ze special zings."

"Oh where have I heard that before? Let me think. Emmanuel said it, Rishi said it, Tony said it, Boris said it, Jacinda said it, and so did Chrystia, Ursula, and even horrid little Theresa. And yet every single one of them profoundly disappointing, I do assure you. Quite without personality, wholly without charm. And, come to think of it, since they're all your little acolytes, Klaus, I really thought you would have trained them better.

"Now, don't get me wrong. It's not that I'm especially fond of Justin. The boy is an absolute dullard, and even dimmer of intellect than all the rest of you, but he is at least accommodating, and that shall suffice for now. Come to think of it, Klaus, do you know who else was in here just the other day offering me 'special zings,' as you put it?"

"I don't know," the man replied wearily.

"Your mate, Charlie boy Windsor! Well, of course, I was so disgusted by the very *idea* of old Sausage Fingers coming anywhere near me that I was tempted to put him out of his misery right there and then. But alas, I'm not permitted to until the Enemy tells me it's time, and apparently, his crimes must be revealed first. Which won't be long now, of course. The Kamloops and Caernarvon revelations are well underway."

"Master, I could bring more evidence against him."

"Down to your last straw now, are you, Klaus? Throwing your friends under the bus to buy yourself a little more time? No, Klaus, there's no need. His fate is sealed... as is yours. Now then, entertaining as this discourse has been, I have other matters to attend to. I'm sure you can understand the burdens of running a global empire. Permit me to dispense with the customary pleasantries such as 'Goodbye' or 'Farewell', much less 'God bless you'. In your case, none of them applies."

"Master! Master!" the man called desperately, but it was all in vain. The red light behind the curtain dimmed to an almost imperceptible glow, and Klaus knew in an instant that all his life's work was for naught. Soon, he would join his mentor Henry in permanent exile from life.

Perhaps that had been the plan all along, to use him and then to discard him as so much medical waste. He would be dead within the day, he was sure of that.

Barely able to stay on his feet, the man shuffled his way back across the checkered tiles and out into the hallway. There, sitting anxiously on a chair beside the wall, was little Justin, ever eager to please. He rose to greet his tutor and extended his hand.

"Hello Klaus," he said with his ingratiating smile. "Good to see you again."

Klaus did not return the gesture, didn't even turn his head to look at the supplicant awaiting his turn to enter the chamber. "Fuck off, you little shit!" he replied, and marched resolutely towards the front door.

Two security men followed him to the vestibule, but Klaus dismissed them with an impatient flick of his hand. Not even an army could protect him now. He put on his coat, eager to cover the expensive robe which now seemed so preposterous, even to his own eyes.

Off came the red shoes too. He didn't even bother undoing the laces this time but held down the back of each shoe with the front of his other foot and hurriedly peeled them off. Cursing under his breath, he picked up his normal shoes from a shoe rack before him and slipped them on. His hands were trembling too much to tie the laces so he left them loose.

He made his way out of the front door and staggered down the front steps of the lodge. The air was cold, and a dim light ahead signalled the beginning of a new day, the close of which he did not expect to see. He took a few deep breaths of the chilly morning air and felt a giddy delight as condensation formed from his breath. These may be his final moments, but at least he would enjoy this last palpable token of life.

His path led him past a garbage bin, where he tossed the red shoes, then towards an old church on his right. It had a sad, dilapidated look to it now. There had been many more funerals there of late, but fewer weddings, and hardly any christenings. Its life was hanging by a thread. He had achieved that much at least, the man thought to himself. Should he go in there now and confess his sins? He laughed at the idea. "Too late for zat now, Klaussy Boy," he chuckled to himself, recalling snippets of the chilling conversation he had just had in the temple lodge.

On the next block, he walked past a school playground where, soon enough, the din of playful children would be heard. “We didn’t kill enough of you,” he whispered to himself.

Immediately, his mind began weaving the old equations, how a rising death count would promote him in the eyes of his collaborators in the secret society, and how the youngest victims would count the most because they were closest to the God he hated. The ones who survived would be trained and traumatized to become wholly indifferent to the suffering of others, a generation of cold-blooded killers, ready to follow orders without question and complete the work of annihilation.

Klaus stopped, placing his hands on the chain-link fence outside the playground, looked in, and sighed. At that moment, a ray of sunlight kissed the side of his face.

“You know this will be the last time you feel the sun, don’t you?” said a voice on his left.

Klaus turned to see who had spoken. A man was standing beside him, wearing a white robe that shimmered in the morning breeze. He too was looking into the playground, but his eyes shone as white fire.

It was time.

January 2024

BOOKS BY A. LEROY (ABDIEL LEROY)

NON-FICTION

KNOW YOUR MEDICAL RIGHTS

Did you know that, under international law, no-one can demand you get a medical test, wear a mask, or have any other medical procedure?

And did you also know that no emergency, even if it threatens the life of a nation, takes away any of your rights? Or that any politician or pundit who attempts to persecute a group based on medical status is committing a Crime Against Humanity?!

Meanwhile, international law also confirms YOUR MEDICAL STATUS IS CONFIDENTIAL, a protection supported by medical codes dating back millennia to the Hippocratic Oath.

Yet governments are not only demanding we hand over this sacred information but are still using it to divide and discriminate, penalizing bodily sovereignty and autonomy, and they are poised to inflict even worse atrocities than they did during 'COVID'.

"I know in my heart that these measures are an atrocity," writes Abdiel LeRoy in the Introduction, "and my spirit rebels against them, but just having that instinct is not enough now. WHAT ARE MY RIGHTS?"

Here is your constitutional Bible, a rebuking voice to tyranny, and a rallying cry for all Mankind.

KNOW YOUR LAWFUL RIGHTS

Not since the days of Noah has Earth witnessed such an all-out assault on life and livelihood as we see today. The false authorities are pursuing their agenda of extermination and enslavement with a ruthlessness most of us could never have imagined.

In this sequel to *Know Your Medical Rights*, Abdiel LeRoy dismantles the lies, programming, and conditioning that have kept us from ourselves. He reminds you who you are, a three-dimensional being standing above the two-dimensional fictions of government, and he empowers you to tear down strongholds of dogma and dictatorship.

"I will show you that all is counterfeit, all theatre," LeRoy writes in the Introduction, "and that counterfeit governments, issuing counterfeit currencies and writing counterfeit legislation masquerading as Law, are wielding counterfeit authority. It's so much easier to refuse and refute that authority when you know its enforcers are beneath you and that they are peddling fictional constructs."

Then, having pierced through the illusions and mind-tricks of tyrants, he lays before you the weapons of True Law you will need to regain your Sovereignty and Birthright. This book will serve you as armour and weapon in the battles ahead.

KNOW YOUR FINANCIAL RIGHTS

Your tax compliance has been funding genocide. Your debt payments are rewarding banks who never lent you anything in the first place. Meanwhile, any digits in your bank account can be seized or freezed at a moment's notice.

The entire financial system has been engineered to extort us, enslave us, and then finally to exterminate us when we've nothing left to give. It's time to tear it down and stop funding our demise, and it's time to transact in ways that tyrants can not monitor, surveil, and control.

Know Your Financial Rights is the final installment of a tyrant-slaying trilogy of constitutional bibles, recalling the mission of Bible prophets who overthrew kings.

Wear this book as a garment of protection, wield it as a spiritual sword, and weaponize it against the legion of traitors now conspiring against us.

THE GOURMET GOSPEL COLLECTION

A Better Eden/ It Was for Freedom/ Foes to Grace

Desperate to escape from an eating disorder, Abdiel went on a quest for "the truth that sets me free," and found it in a rediscovery of Grace—the unmerited favor of God—that church teachings rarely, if ever, reveal.

With the help of great writers, Christian thinkers, and of course the Bible itself, he returns to an Eden of the mind that predates the command, 'Do not...', and where sin is neither possible nor perceived.

DUELING THE DRAGON COLLECTION

Five Memoirs About Living and Working in China

A wide-eyed expat is detained by Beijing cops and told to sign a false confession. Will he make it out of China alive? *Dueling the Dragon* is a great adventure story, but *this* one just happens to be true!

With a journalist's eye and lively wit, LeRoy's memoirs expose the deep levels of corruption tearing at China's social fabric.

MY PORTABLE PARADISE

Transform Your Life Through House Sitting

Tired of burning bitter hours in a toxic job? Tired of the same old routine? Tired of the stress and hassle of paying rent, or a mortgage? Then house sitting may be for you.

From a beach house in Costa Rica, this veteran house sitter and author welcomes you to share in the joys and blessings he has received.

Whether you're a 'digital nomad' looking for adventure, retired and seeking a change of scenery, or just looking for a simpler life, you'll find gentle guidance in this book. And... it might just change your life!

POETRY COLLECTIONS

WELL VERSED

To Shakespeare, Poets, and the Performing Arts

Dante is famous. He imagined Hell,
A plain of burning flakes and sulphurous smell,
Pour souls afflicted in a sorry state,
And names the enemies he loves to hate.

But he's no match for Milton's inspiration,
No poet greater in imagination.
Yet Shakespeare most gets ink within these pages.
'Twas he who said, "Our praises are our wages!"

VERSES VERSUS EMPIRE
I—The Bush Era

It's Judgment Day, and George W. Bush strides confidently towards the throne of God. How will the Almighty respond? Find out in this work of devastating satire.

From Bush through Obama to Trump, LeRoy charts an epic course through the inferno of U.S. politics, exposing the fraud and folly of empire and its rulers.

VERSES VERSUS EMPIRE
II—The Obama Era

As the late historian Howard Zinn said, "There have only been a handful of people who use their wit to take down the pretensions of the high and mighty."

Here is one of them, a resounding voice for our times, an offering of hope and beauty rising from the ashes of a broken political system, a creation of unprecedented literary power. Witness herein that the pen really *is* mightier than the sword!

VERSES VERSUS EMPIRE

III—The Trump Era

The intellectuals of this dangerous age,
However eloquent, however sage,
Indicting empire with insightful prose,
Have not yet healed the nation's woes.

To tear down strongholds of the powers-that-be
Who give lip service to Democracy,
A poet of prophetic voice steps forward
To prove the pen is mightier than the sword!

THE VERSES VERSUS EMPIRE COLLECTION

Poetry and Prose on Three Imperial Presidencies

2001-2021

Through three imperial presidencies
The poet cries, voice in the wilderness,
Reed swaying in the wind,[i] *a bruisèd reed,*[ii]
His motion stirred to music,
Daring to see and state the obvious,
Decry hypocrisy, prophetically to see
Not just the future but the now,
The awful now and make some sense of it,
The world a stage on which plays out
Congressional pantomime, a knot
Unable to untie itself. The blood
Of innocents cries out to Heaven where
These incensed lines as incense burn
With hate of Hate and hope of Hope.

EPIC POETRY

(FICTION IN VERSE)

ELIJAH

A Fictional Reinvention of the Great Prophet's Life
in an Epic Poem

He called down fire and false prophets slew,
He raised the dead, conversed with angels, flew
To Heaven in a chariot of fire
And fled from Jezebel's murderous ire.

But there is more, O so much more to tell,
Of meeting Moses and a dragon's spell,
Shapeshifting goddesses at Cherith Brook.
Such wonders will unfold within this book!

OBAMA'S DREAM

The Journey That Changed the World

This sordid theatre we call politics
Is full of lies and dirty tricks,
But what if angels came into the fray
To challenge presidents and what they say?

And what if one appeared before God's throne
Where wicked schemes of men are overthrown
And Satan tried a victim to condemn?
This book turns upside-down the world of men!

THE EPICS COLLECTION

Obama's Dream, Elijah, Jezebel's Lament

It is an age-old struggle, that between
The earthly power of presidents and kings
Encountering divine power, wonders seen
When prophets pray. This theme the author brings

In reinvention of the Bible tales,
Ascents to Heaven, wondrous revelation,
Shapeshifting goddesses in his portrayals,
Joined by the author's audiobook narrations.

FICTION

JEZEBEL'S LAMENT

A Defense of Reputation, a Denouncement of the prophets Elijah and Elisha

In this companion piece to *Elijah*, Israel's tyrant queen tells her side of the story and why she so detests that "unkempt fire-and-brimstone hairy hermit" who prophesies dogs shall eat her corpse.

"Yes, I had to get rid of some inconvenient men of God along the way, and a stubborn wine producer, but in all this I did only what a queen *must* do in such circumstances to protect herself, to safeguard her family and the royal line."

You will hear of trysts and treason in this witty rendering by Abdiel LeRoy.

THE CHRISTMAS TREE
A Tale of Divine Awakening

A tree is torn from his forest home and all that he loves, but there is courage in the heart of a little boy to protect his belovèd tree.

The author dreamt up this story from witnessing Christmas trees being abandoned on city sidewalks, but here his invention of a magical journey for one such tree will transport you through time and space and otherworldly encounter, even to the throne of God!

THE PRINCE'S OATH
A Tale From Afghanistan

An innocent man must lose his freedom, an innocent girl must yield her virginity, in this traditional tale from an era of kings.

From bandit attacks in a forest to treacherous plots at court, love will undergo many trials with the Almighty's help, even if it comes in the form of a cheeky little mouse!

THE CHRISTIAN REVERIES COLLECTION

The Christmas Tree/ The Prince's Oath/ Obama's Dream

You'll know a tree according to its fruit,
Three golden branches with one holy root,
The Good Book's inspiration running through,
This trinity uplifting hearts anew.

Not 'R'-rated as the Epics Collection,
These tales are more of a 'PG' selection,
But still have magic, shapeshifters, and all
Those elements mythology recalls.

NOTES

Introduction to 'Know Your Medical Rights'

i. Addressing the Belmarsh Tribunal that examined state crimes against Julian Assange, Oct. 22, 2021.
ii. *Matthew* 17:20.
iii. Shakespeare, *Hamlet*, III.ii.
iv. At the time of going to press, the first novel in this series, titled *The Lamp of Darkness*, was free in eBook version at various on-line retailers.

Poetry Collections

i. Matthew 11:7.
ii. Matthew 12:20.

www.ingramcontent.com/pod-product-compliance
Ingram Content Group UK Ltd.
Pitfield, Milton Keynes, MK11 3LW, UK
UKHW022022041026
15591UKWH00012B/442

9 781917 073165